DIAGNOSTIC
Picture Tests in Clinical Medicine

2

G S J Chessell, Dip Ed Tech.
Coordinator, Medical Learning Resources Group, University of Aberdeen

M J Jamieson, MRCP
Lecturer, Department of Therapeutics and Clinical Pharmacology, University of Aberdeen

R A Morton, MSc
Director, Department of Medical Illustration, University of Aberdeen

J C Petrie, FRCP
Reader, Department of Therapeutics and Clinical Pharmacology, University of Aberdeen; Honorary Consultant Physician, Aberdeen Teaching Hospitals.

H M A Towler, MRCP
Lecturer, Department of Medicine, University of Aberdeen.

Wolfe Publishing Ltd

Published by Wolfe Medical Publications Ltd 1984
Printed by Grafos, Arte Sobre Papel, Barcelona, Spain
Volume 1 ISBN 0 7234 0848 3
Volume 2 ISBN 0 7234 0849 1
Volume 3 ISBN 0 7234 0850 5
Volume 4 ISBN 0 7234 0851 3

Reprinted 1985, 1987, 1989, 1991, 1992

For a full list of Wolfe Medical Atlases, plus forthcoming titles and details of our surgical, dental and veterinary Atlases, please write to Wolfe Publishing Limited,
Brook House,
2-16 Torrington Place
London WC1E 7LT

PREFACE

This is volume two of a four-volume series. The aim is to test diagnostic skills over a wide range of clinical problems. Questions which may feature in examinations or in clinical practice are posed in an attempt to stimulate the undergraduate or postgraduate reader to undertake further reading.

The pictures in this new series have been selected from the clinical slide library in the Department of Medical Illustration, University of Aberdeen. The books have been produced against a background of experience gained over the last 10 years in the compilation for local use of over 2,000 self-assessment examples. The local exercise was coordinated through the Medical Learning Resources Group of the Faculty of Medicine, University of Aberdeen, in collaboration with many of the clinicians in the Aberdeen Teaching Hospitals.

We hope that the books will be of interest to all who are committed to their own continuing medical education. We would welcome comment on individual questions and answers.

GSJC, MJJ, RAM, JCP, HMAT.

Although numbering is sequential, each volume in the series is unique, containing a balanced selection of diagnostic examples, and thus may be used independently.

ACKNOWLEDGEMENTS

We wish to acknowledge the invaluable contribution of Dr Anthony Hedley, now Professor of Community Medicine, University of Glasgow, who was the instigator of the self-assessment programme on which these books are based. We would also like to acknowledge the cooperation of all patients, secretarial and technical staff, in particular the staff of the Department of Medical Illustration, who have contributed in one way or another to the preparation of these volumes, and Mrs Margaret Doverty who typed the manuscript.

We would particularly like to thank the following colleagues for contributing material for the books:

Dr D R Abramovich, Mr A Adam, Mr A K Ah-See, Dr D J G Bain, Dr L S Bain, Dr K Bartlett, Dr A P Bayliss, Dr B Bennett, Miss F M Bennett, Dr P Best, Dr P D Bewsher, Mr C Birchall, Mr C T Blaiklock, Dr L J Borthwick, Mr P L Brunnen, Dr P W Brunt, Dr J Calder, Professor A G M Campbell, Dr B Carrie, Dr P Carter, Dr G R D Catto, Mr R B Chesney, Dr N Clark, Mr P B Clarke, Mr A I Davidson, Dr R J L Davidson, Dr A A Dawson, Mr W B M Donaldson, Professor A S Douglas, Dr A W Downie, Dr C J Eastmond, Mr J Engeset, Dr N Edward, Dr J K Finlayson, Dr J R S Finnie, Mr A V Foote, Dr N G Fraser, Mr R J A Fraser, Dr J A R Friend, Dr D B Galloway, Mr J M C Gibson, Dr D Hadley, Dr J E C Hern, Dr A W Hutcheon, Dr T A Jeffers, Dr A W Johnston, Mr P F Jones, Dr A C F Kenmure, Mr I R Kernohan, Dr A S M Khir, Mr J Kyle, Dr J S Legge, Mr McFadzean, Dr E McKay, Mr J McLauchlan, Mr K A McLay, Professor M MacLeod, Dr R A Main, Mr Mather, Mr N A Matheson, Mr J D B Miller, Mr S S Miller, Mr K L G Mills, Dr N A G Mowat, Mr I F K Muir, Dr L E Murchison, Mr W J Newlands, Mr J G Page, Professor R Postlethwaite, Dr J M Rawles, Mr P K Ray, Mr C R W Rayner, Professor A M Rennie, Mr A G R Rennie, Dr J A N Rennie, Dr O J Robb, Dr H S Ross, Dr G Russell, Dr D S Short, Dr P J Smail, Dr C C Smith, Professor G Smith, Dr L Stankler, Mr J H Steyn, Professor J M Stowers, Dr G H Swapp, Mr J Wallace, Professor W Walker, Dr S J Watt, Dr J Weir, Dr J Webster, Dr M I White, Dr F W Wigzell, Dr M J Williams, Mr L C Wills, Dr L A Wilson, Mr H A Young.

195 and 196 This mentally subnormal patient has recently had a first grand mal seizure. The unusual appearance of his finger nail led to close examination of the optic fundi.

a What abnormality is seen in the nail?
b What abnormality is seen adjacent to the optic disc?
c What unusual cause of epilepsy do these suggest?
d What is the risk that his younger sister is also affected?

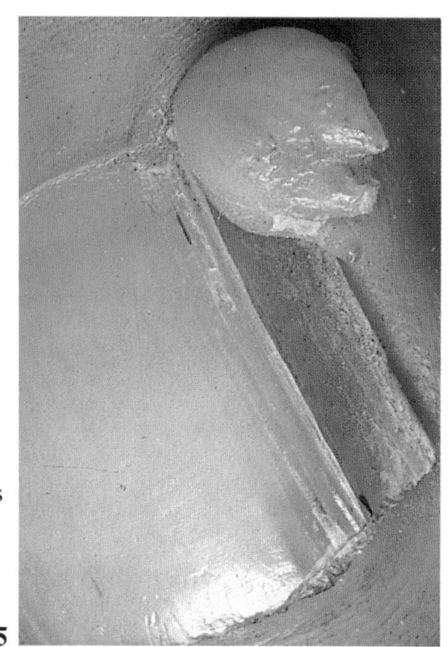

195

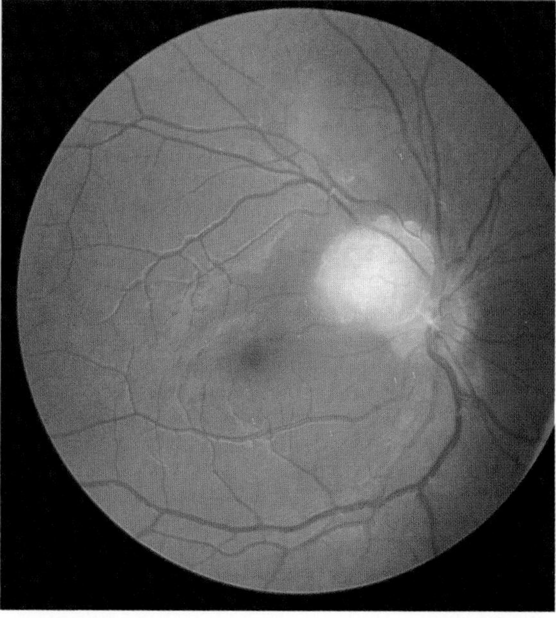

196

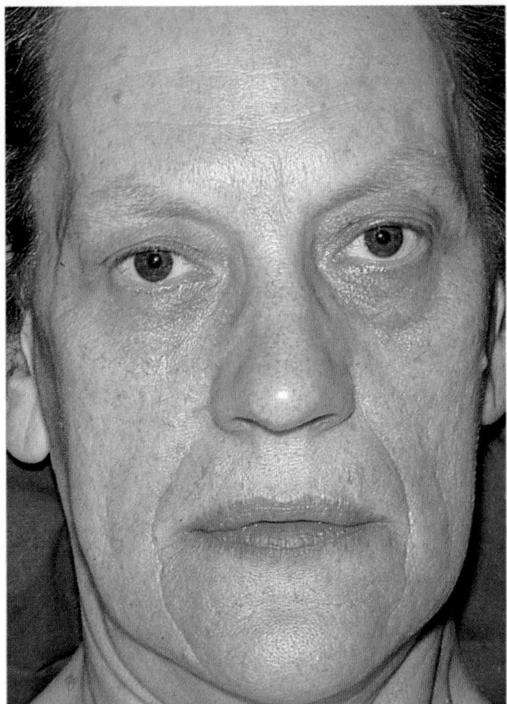

197

197

This patient complains of tiredness and excessive sweating.

a What diagnosis is suggested by her facial appearance?

b What treatments are available for this condition?

c Which radiological finding is most important in determining the type of treatment employed?

198

This thirty-two year old male presented with accelerated hypertension.

a Name the structures labelled 1-5 seen on CT scan through the upper abdomen.

b What is the likely diagnosis?

198

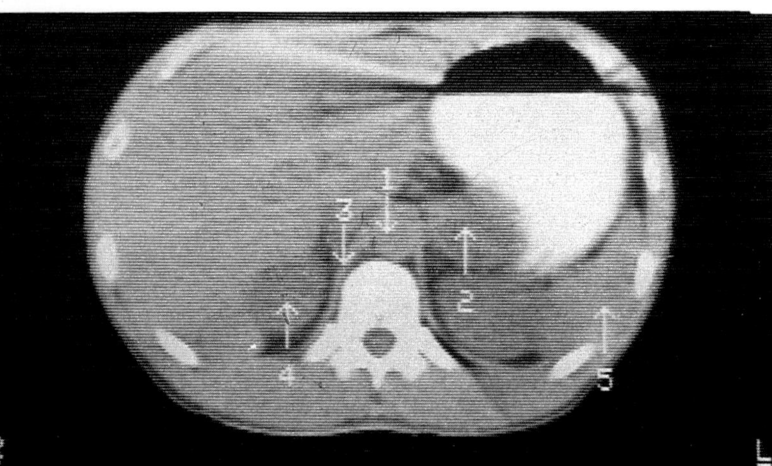

199

This twenty-two year old female patient has become increasingly breathless after taking aspirin for period pains.

a What principal radiological abnormality is seen?

b What is the likely diagnosis?

c Is she more likely to complain of difficulty breathing in or breathing out?

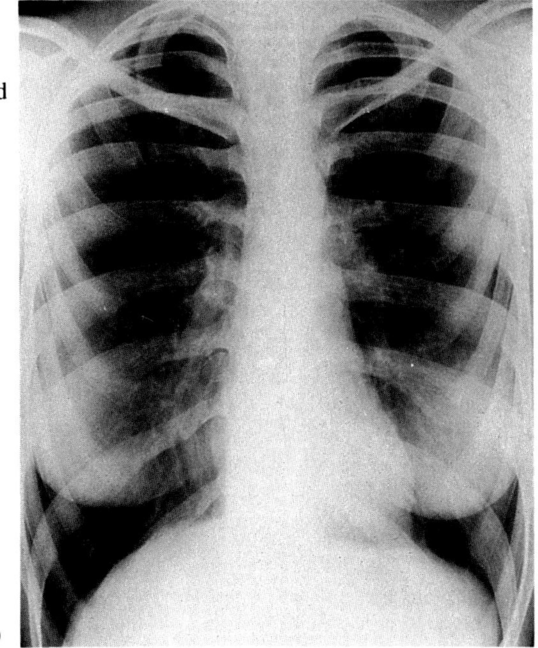

199

200

This is the peripheral blood film of a fifty-six year old man who presented with tiredness and a sensation of abdominal fullness. 15 cm splenomegaly was noted. His haemoglobin was 9.5 g/dl, white cell count 130 x 10^9/1, and platelets 600 x 10^9/1.

a What diagnosis does the film suggest?

b Name three investigations performed on peripheral blood which may help establish the diagnosis.

c Name four drugs employed in the management of this disease.

200

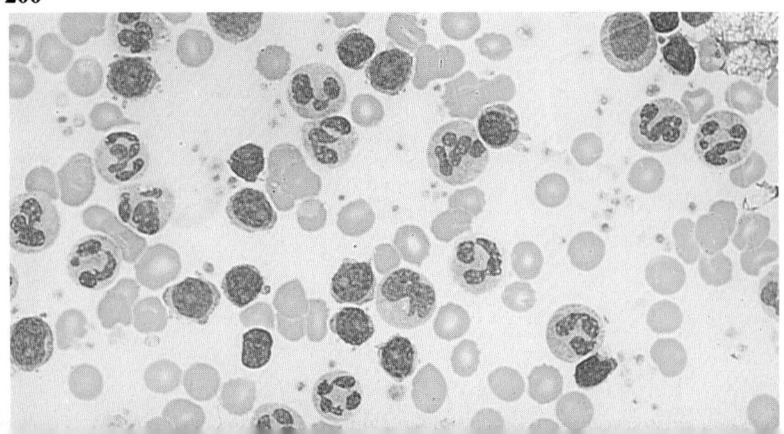

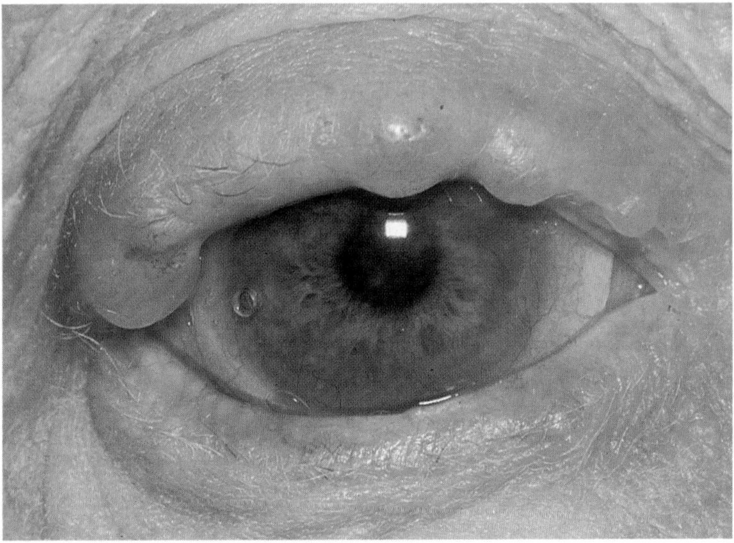

201 This woman has ocular cicatrical pemphigoid. **201**

a What is the main complication of this condition?
b What would immunofluorescence studies of a skin biopsy show?
c Is this associated with underlying malignancy?

202 This driver of an articulated lorry complains of chest pain.

a What is the diagnosis?
b When should he return to driving his lorry?

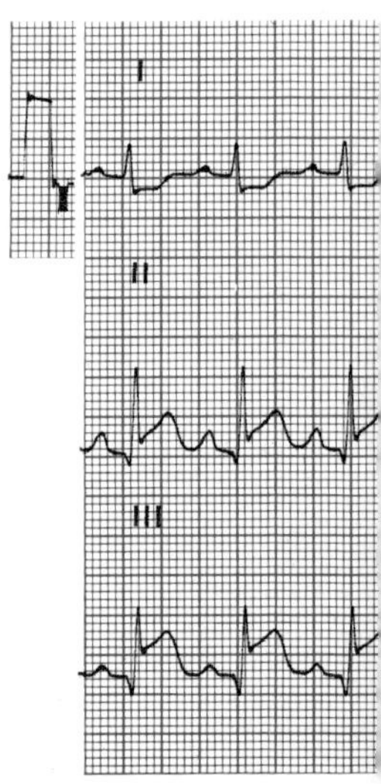

203

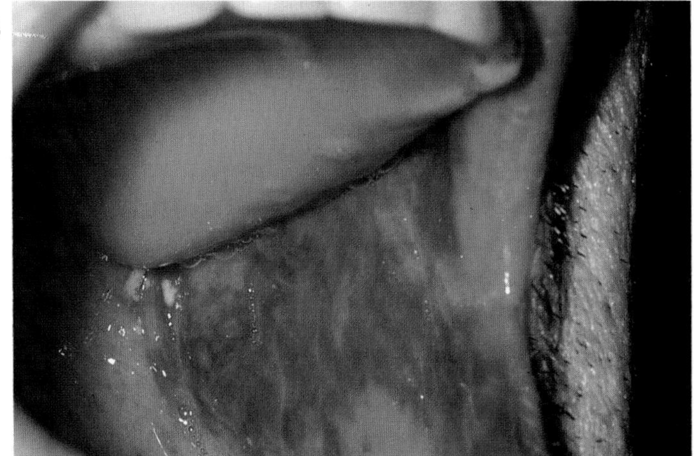

203

This forty-five year old man presented with a short history of increasing muscle weakness, weight loss and ankle swelling. He was unable to rise from a chair without using his arms. His blood pressure was 180/110 mm Hg. sitting.

a What is the likely diagnosis?
b Where is the likely site of the underlying lesion?
c What electrolyte abnormality may be present?
d Which investigations may help establish the diagnosis?

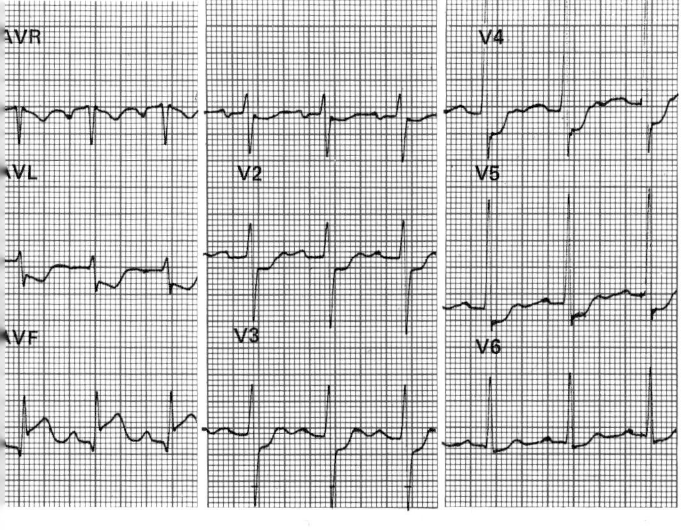

202

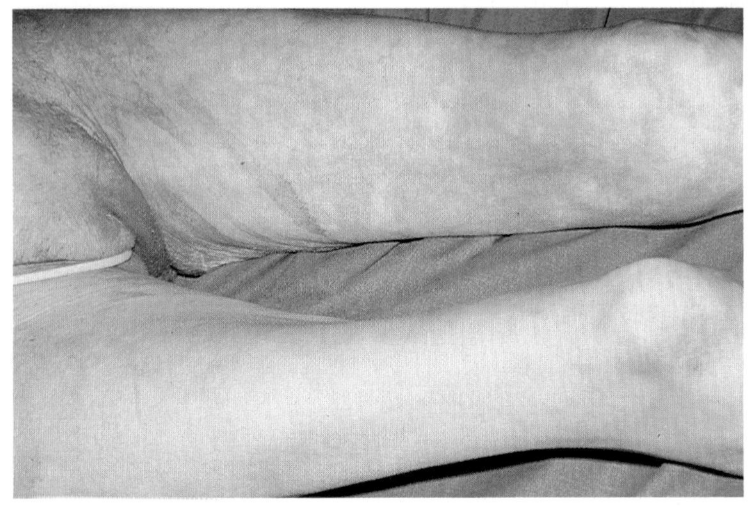

204

205

204
This patient has been in hospital for three months following a stroke. She has longstanding mitral valve disease. Four hours ago she complained of pain and coldness affecting her left leg.

a What is the likely diagnosis?
b What is the most likely origin of this problem?
c What disorder of cardiac rhythm would you expect to find?

205
This female patient is a recent immigrant into the United Kingdom from India.

a What bony abnormality is seen in her x-ray?
b In which other sites are these typically seen?
c What metabolic disorder do these indicate?

206 This patient complains of severe generalised pruritus, worst when in bed at night.

a What is the most likely diagnosis?

b In which sites should the causative agent be sought?

c How is the diagnosis confirmed?

207 This child has always been prone to chest infections. Her height is consistently below the third centile for her age. Recently, for the first time, her fingers have been seen to be intermittently cyanosed. A pansystolic murmur is audible at the left sternal edge. E.C.G. shows tall P waves in standard lead II and dominant R waves in leads V_1 to V_3.

a What is the most likely diagnosis?

b Why is she cyanosed?

c What abnormalities in haemodynamics and in oxygen saturation would you expect to find at cardiac catheterisation?

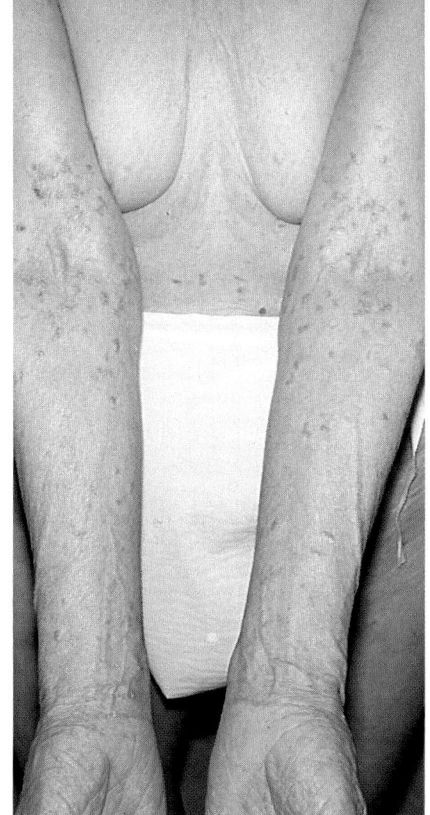

206

207

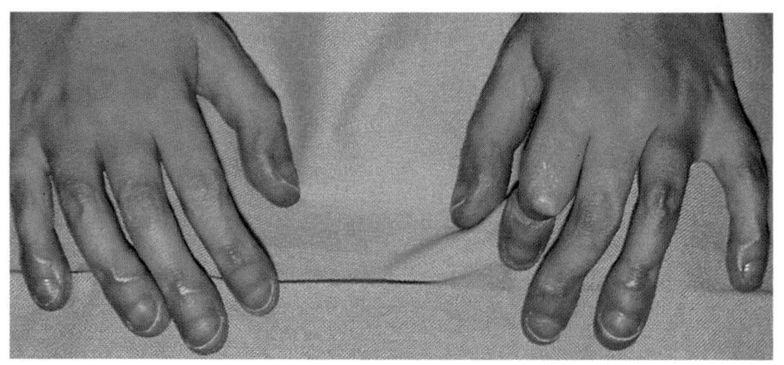

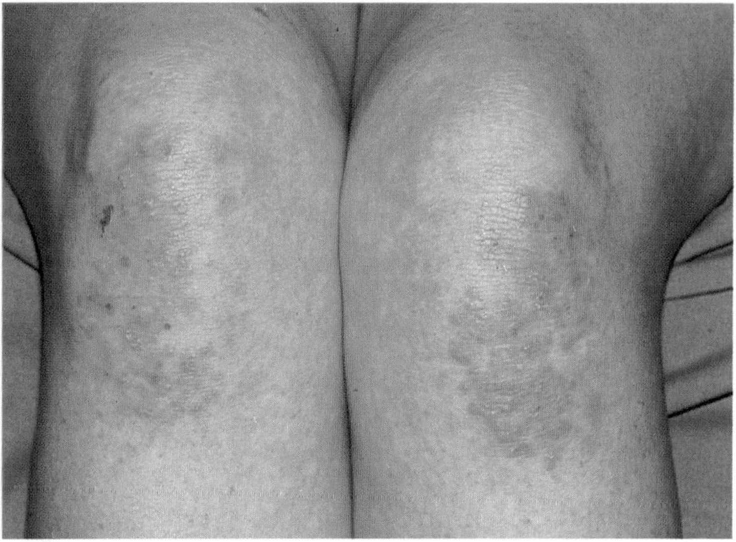

208

209 a What name is given to this infection?
b What is the infecting organism?
c What is its usual origin?

209

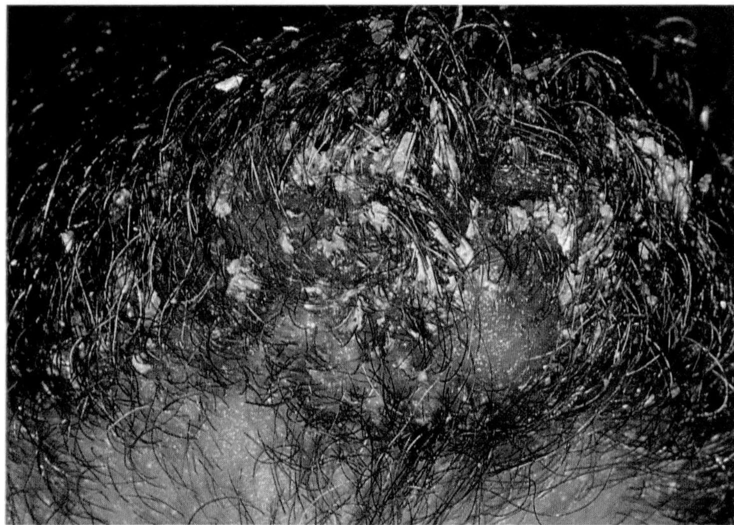

208
This patient complains of an intensely itchy skin rash. On specific questioning she admits to chronic mild diarrhoea, the stools on occasion being difficult to flush.
a What name is given to the skin rash?
b What is likely to be the cause of her abdominal symptoms?
c What two forms of treatment may improve the skin rash?

210
a What name is given to the lesion seen on the right side of this patient's tongue?
b What is its significance?

211
This Asian patient was asked to look to his left.
a What abnormality of eye movement is shown?
b What is the cranial nerve lesion involved?

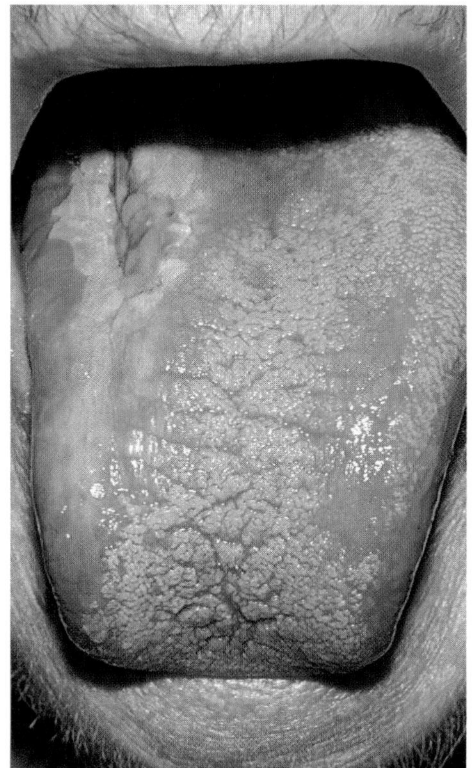

210

211

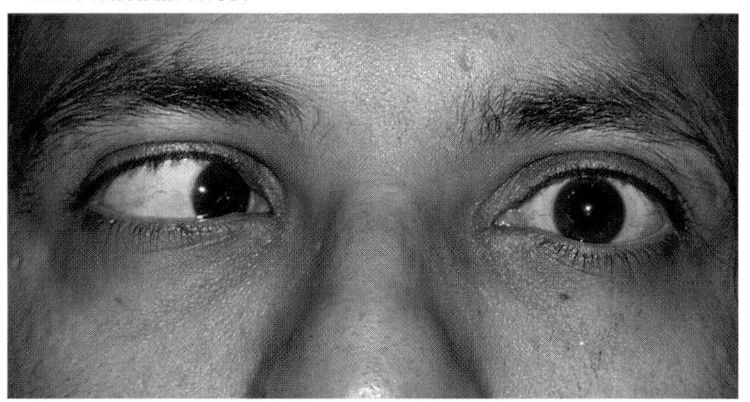

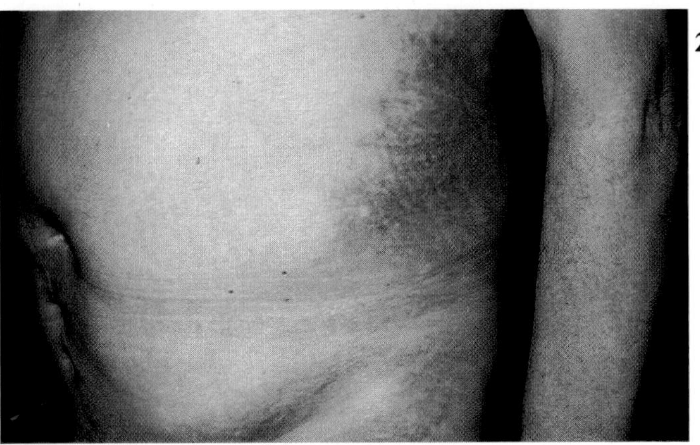

212

212
This patient presents with acute onset spontaneous back pain.
a Which two eponymous signs are present?
b Which diagnoses should be considered?

213
a Which two abnormalities are seen here?
b What is the most likely underlying disorder?
c List four other stigmata of this disorder which may be observed in the hands.

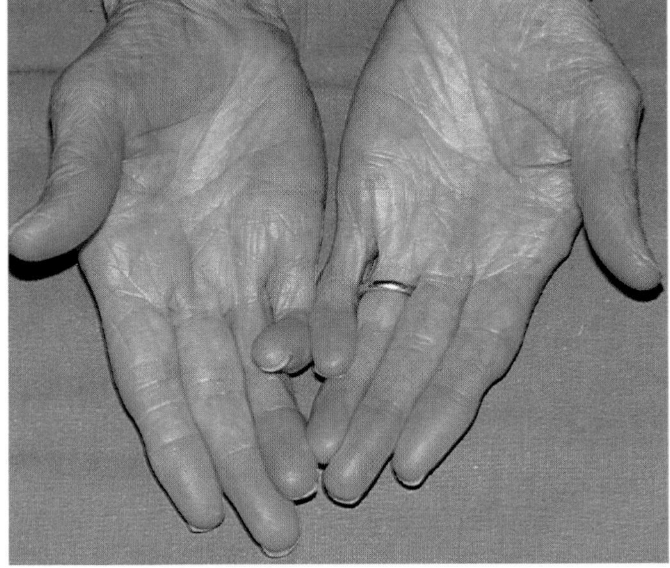

213

214
This patient complains of sudden visual loss in this eye.
What abnormality is seen in this peripheral area of the fundus?

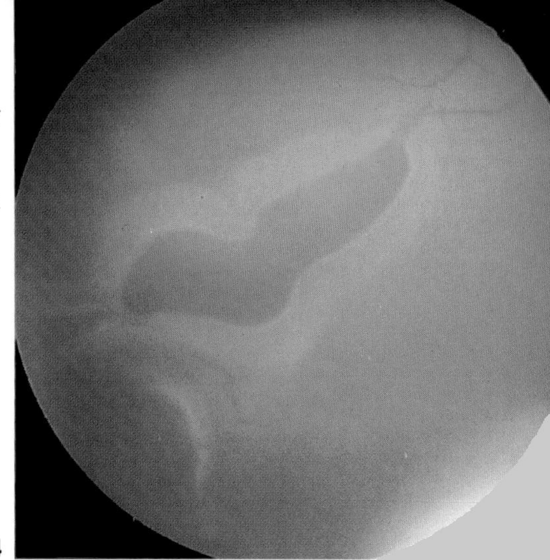

214

215
This male child falls frequently and finds running difficult. There is a family history of similar problems.

a What muscular abnormality is shown?
b What is the likely diagnosis?
c What eponym is used to describe the characteristic manoeuvre by which such children stand up from lying prone?

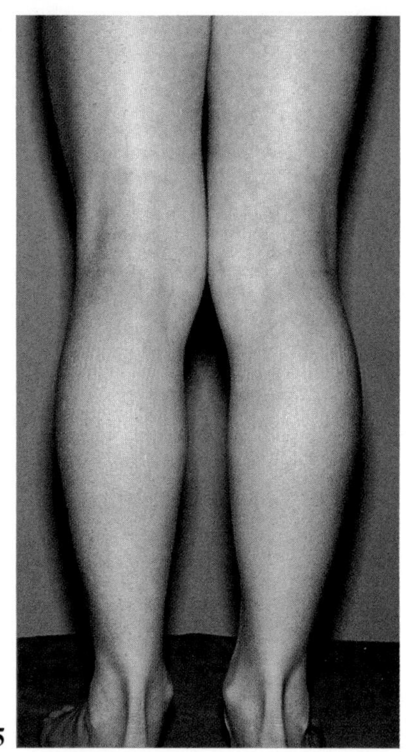

215

216 and 217 This patient has recently developed dysphagia.

a What principal abnormalities are seen in
   i) the head?
   ii) the hands?

b What is the underlying diagnosis?

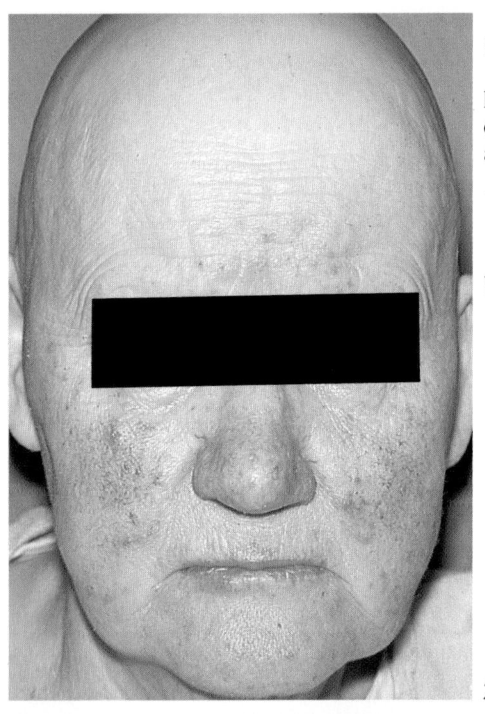

216

217

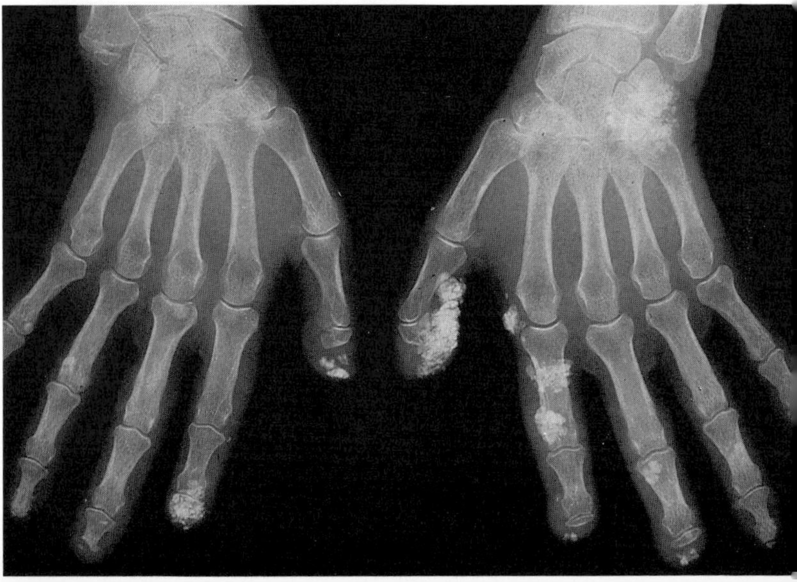

218

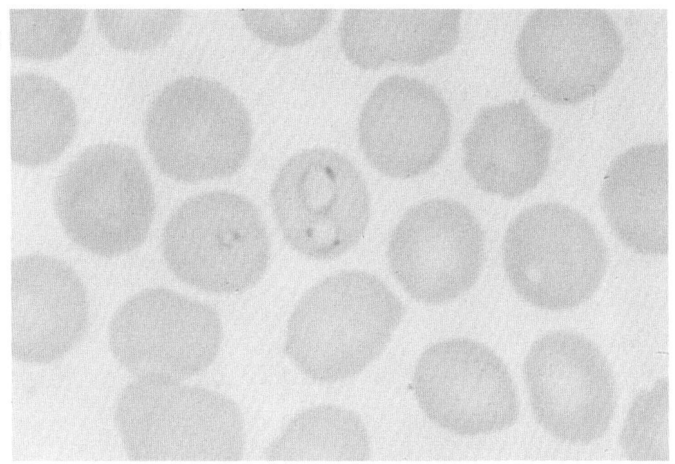

218 This oilworker recently returned from Thailand, having taken chloroquine anti-malarial prophylaxis. He complained of fever, headache, and widespread arthralgia.

a What abnormality is seen on this thin blood film?
b What immediate therapy is indicated?
c What prophylaxis would have been appropriate?

219

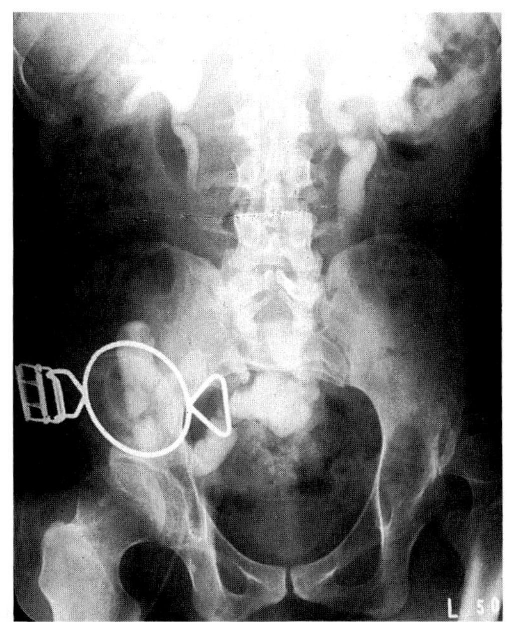

219

a List four abnormalities visible on this child's intravenous pyelogram.
b What electrolyte disturbances are typical of the urinary abnormality?
c Would you expect to find an anion gap?

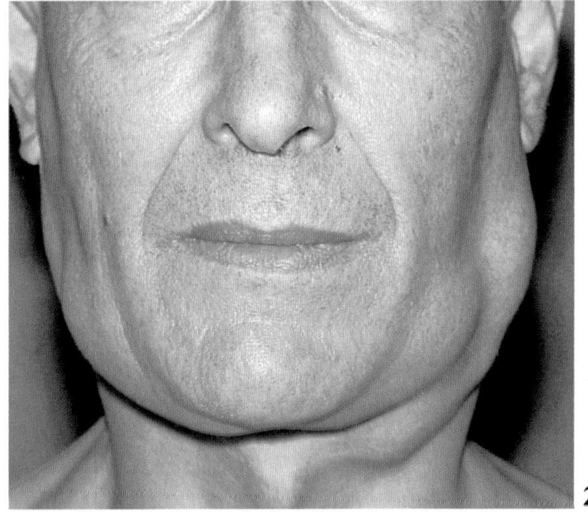
220

220
This man's white cell count is 78 x 10^9/1 with a differential count of 3% neutrophils and 97% lymphocytes.
a What is the likely diagnosis?
b Name three ways in which this condition may give rise to jaundice.
c What is the immediate effect of prednisolone on the white cell count?

221
a What name is given to this lesion?
b What treatment is necessary?

221
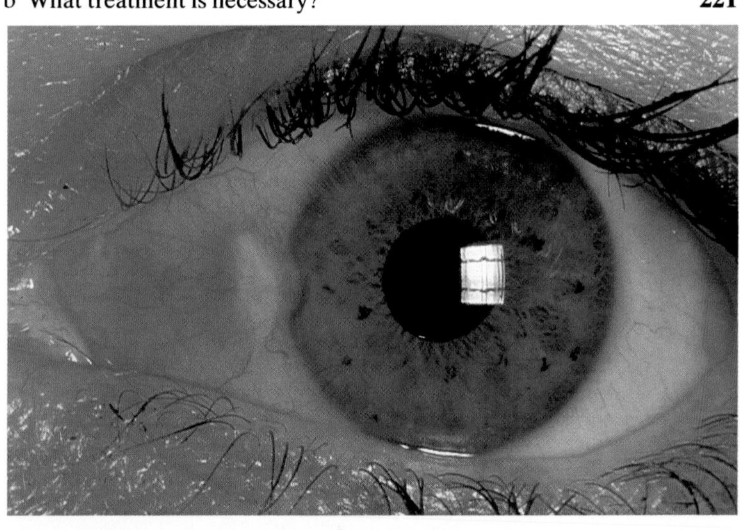

222

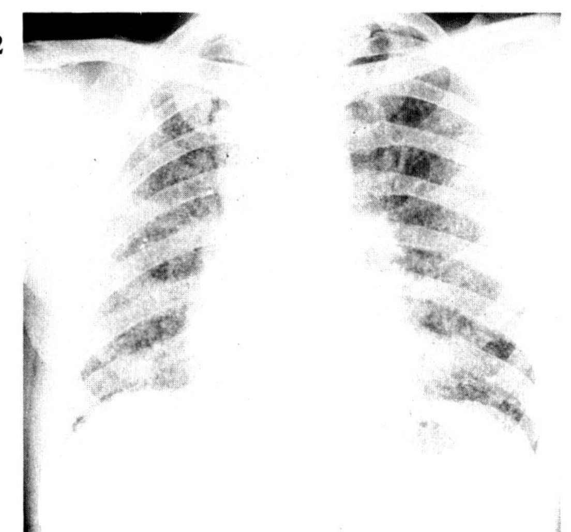

222 and 223

This patient complains of non-productive cough of three months duration.

a What principal abnormality is seen on chest x-ray.
b Describe the abnormality seen on skull x-ray?
c What condition is suggested by these appearances?

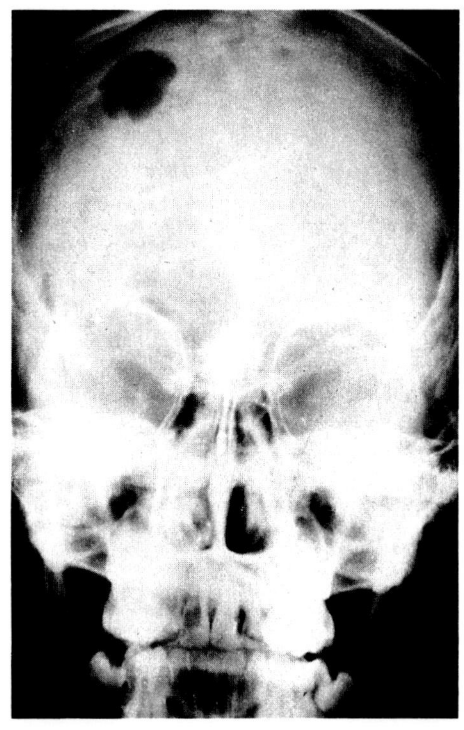

223

224
This patient is on long-term treatment for a psychotic disorder. He presents with a gradual increase in the number of these lesions on his left shin.

a What is the most likely cause of these lesions?
b What is the typical distribution of such lesions?

225
This patient has rheumatoid arthritis.

a What abnormality is seen at the elbow?
b What two simple tests are useful in indicating the nature of the swelling?

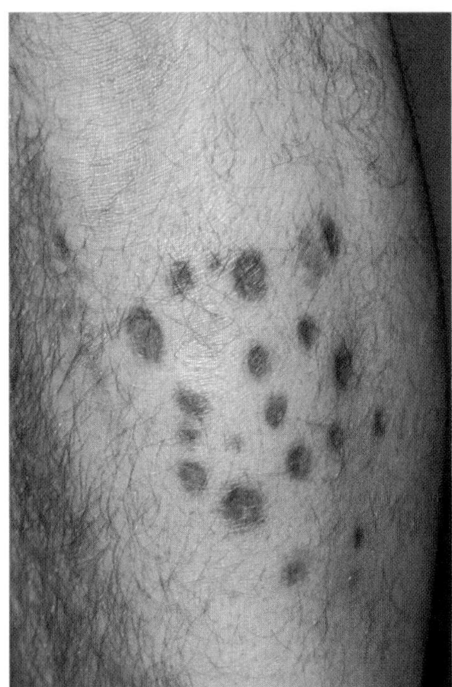
224

225
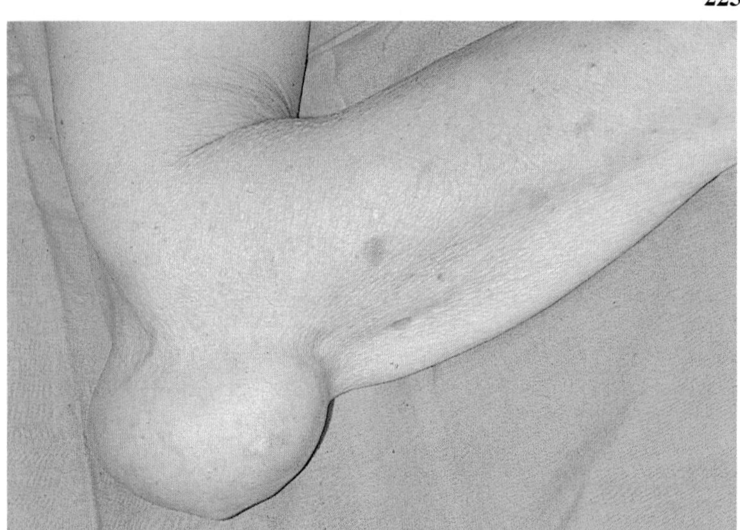

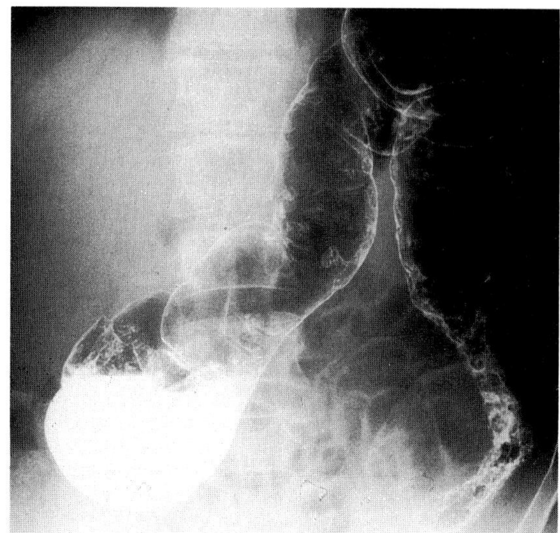

226

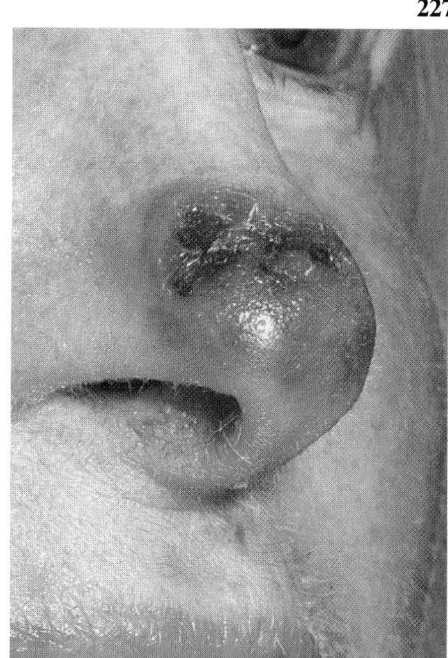

227

226 and 227

This patient suffers from recurrent bloody diarrhoea. The lesion seen on her nose began as a tender red nodule, which became bluish before ulcerating. The appearance has changed little over the past four weeks.

a List four abnormal features seen on double contrast barium enema.
b What is the most likely diagnosis?
c What name is given to the skin condition?
d List three other causes of this skin disorder.

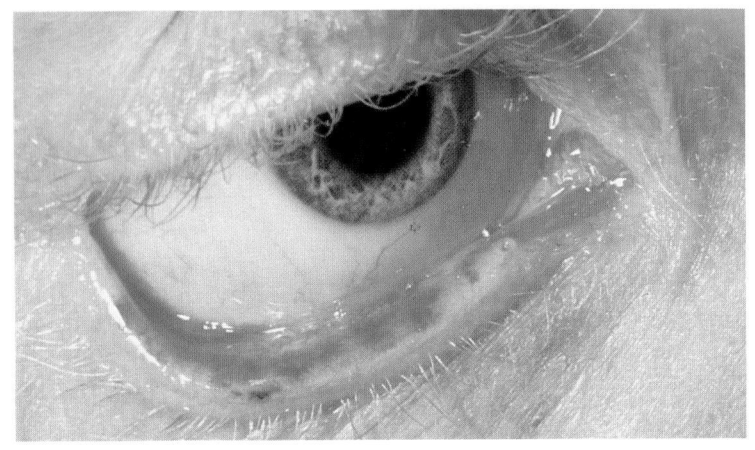

228

228 and 229 This man presented with weight loss, low grade fever and a cardiac murmur. Blood cultures grew streptococcus bovis.
- a What is the diagnosis?
- b What is the likely source of this organism?
- c What is unusual about its antibiotic sensitivity?
- d With what condition is this infection associated?

229

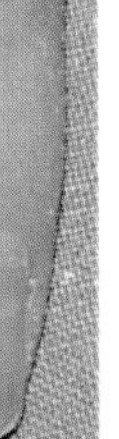

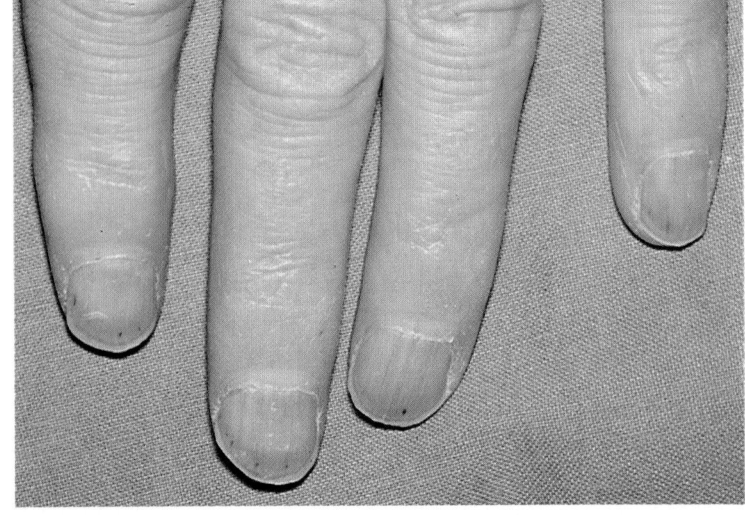

230

a What name is given to this appearance?

b Which organisms may be involved?

c What other condition is usually present?

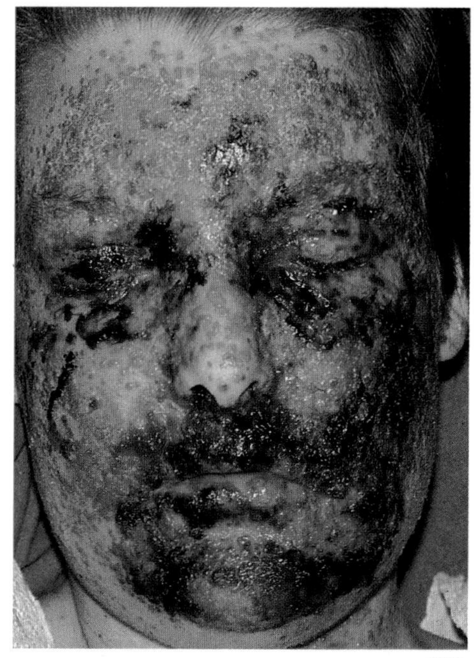

230

231 a Describe the abnormalities present.

b What is the likely aetiology?

c What is the most likely predisposing factor in this case?

231

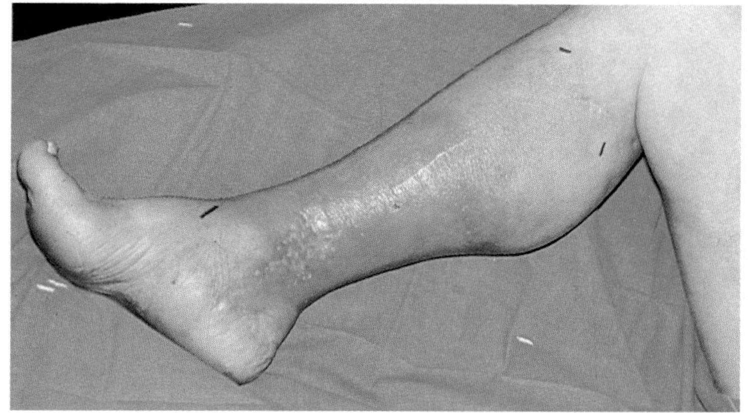

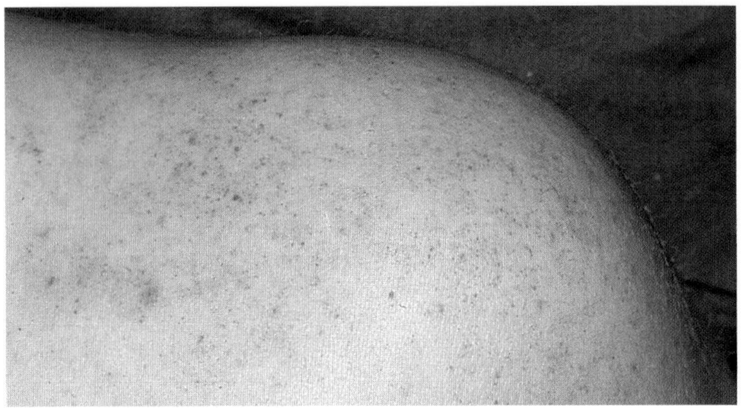

232

233

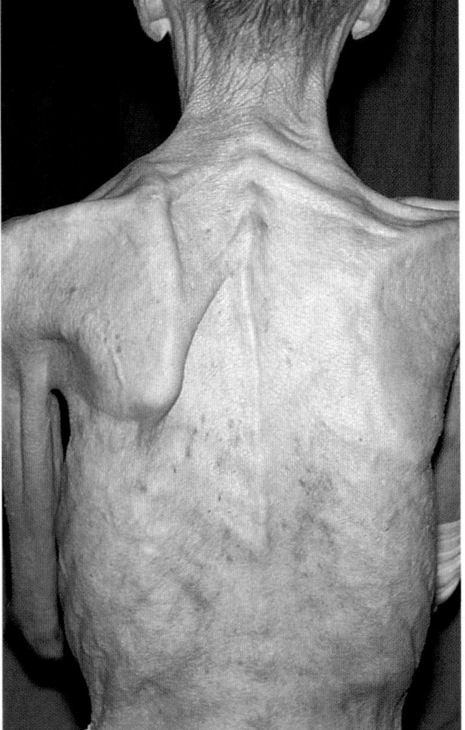

232
This young patient has become confused and aggressive shortly after his admission to a casualty ward.
What is the cause of his confusion?

233
This cachectic patient has an intrathoracic neoplasm.
a What neurological abnormality is shown?
b Which muscle is affected?
c In this case, what is the likely underlying cause?

234
This patient complained of recurring inflammation of his ears and nose and occasional 'rheumatic' pains in his chest, accompanied by fever. On several occasions, he had been treated for erysipelas with benzyl penicillin, with no response.

a What is the diagnosis?
b How may the diagnosis be established?
c Which complications may be life-threatening?

235
This immigrant patient complains of recurrent colicky abdominal pain and constipation.

a What abnormality is shown?
b What is the diagnosis?
c Give four other clinical features of this disorder.

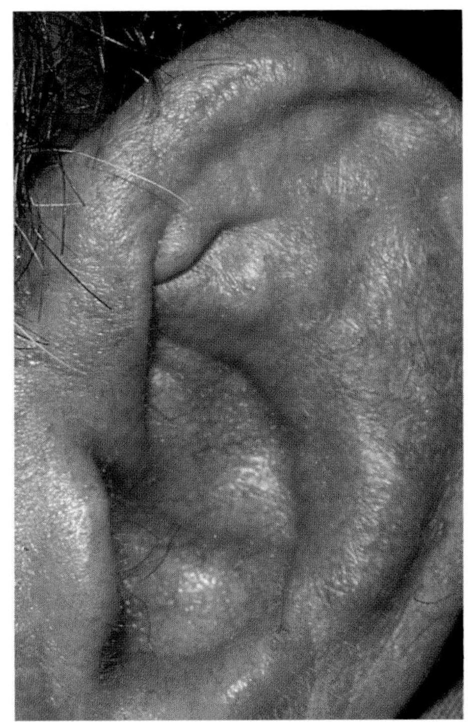

234

235

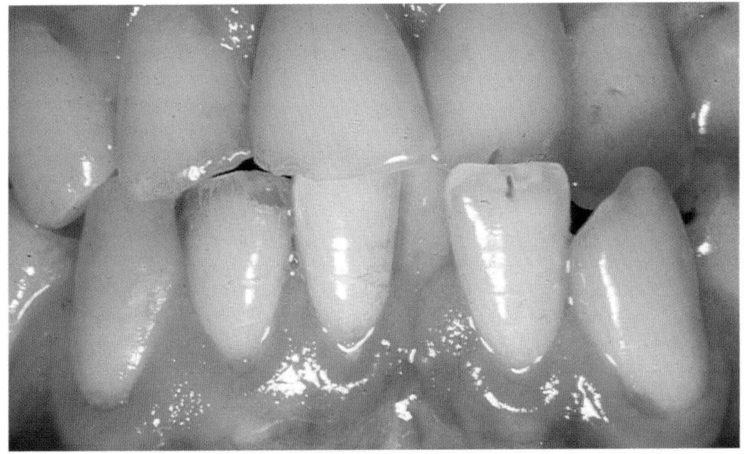

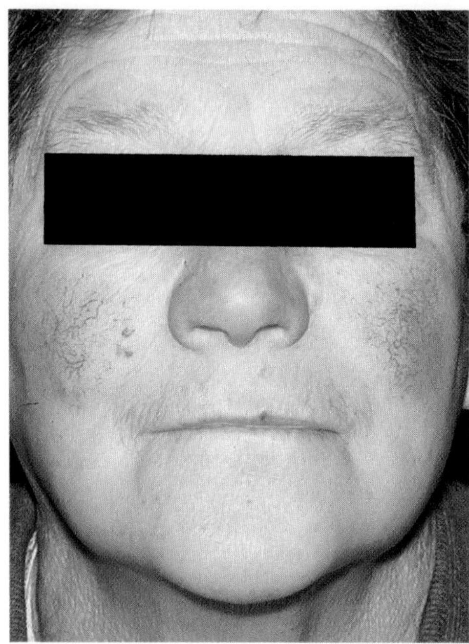

236

236
This woman presented with tiredness and increasing weight. Laboratory findings included a macrocytic anaemia which showed no improvement following folic acid or vitamin B12 administration.

a What is the cause of her symptoms?
b How should her anaemia be treated?

237
This patient is an insulin-dependent diabetic. What are the lesions seen in the periphery of the fundus?

237

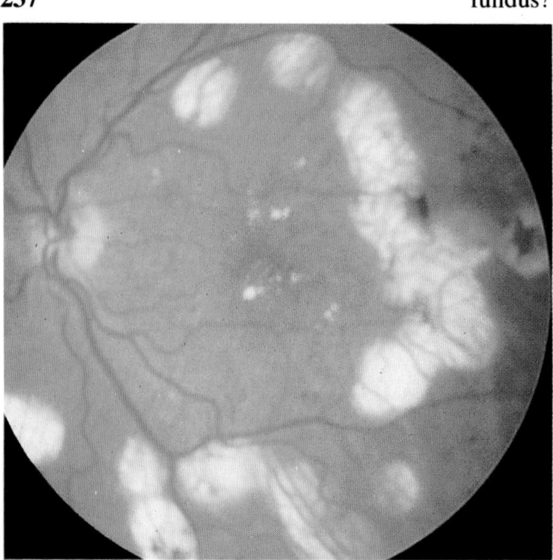

238

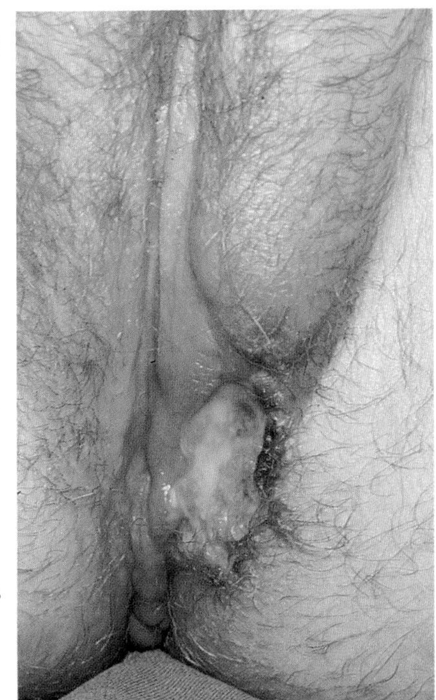

238 and 239 This woman presented with recurrent painful ulcers as demonstrated.

a What is the likely diagnosis?

b What other organ is classically involved?

c What laboratory test is diagnostic of this condition?

d Which sex is more likely to be affected?

239

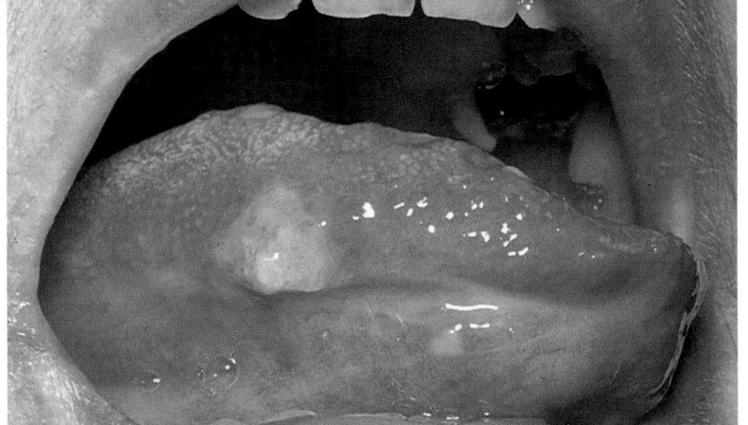

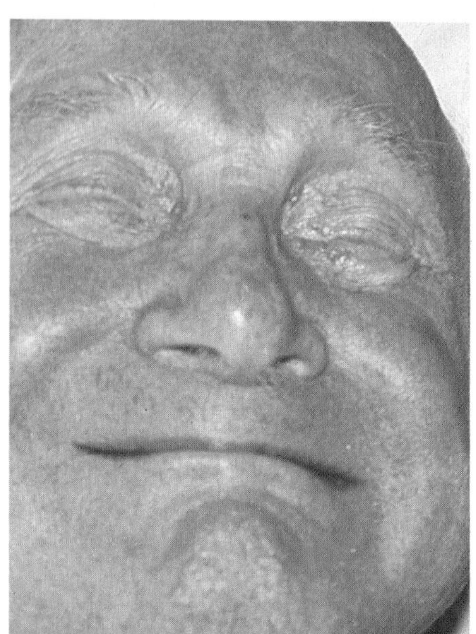

240

This 'smile' is involuntary.

a What name is given to this appearance?
b What is its cause?
c Suggest two drugs which may give rise to a similar appearance

240

241

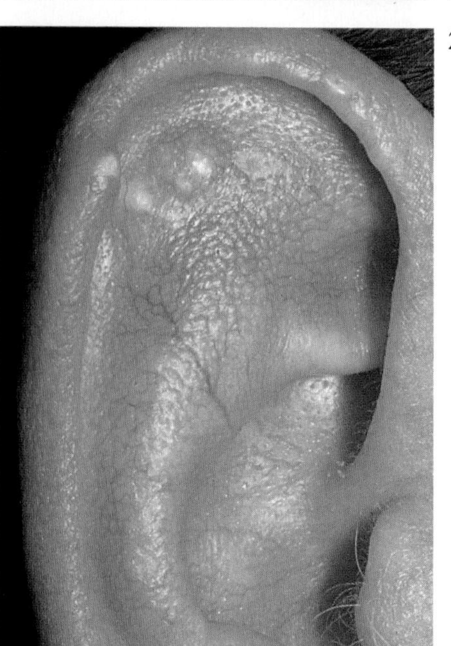

241

This patient suffers from recurrent episodes of joint pain and swelling.

a What are these lesions?
b Which two investigations would be most helpful in establishing the diagnosis?

242 This girl presented at the age of eighteen years with primary amenorrhoea and small stature. Neurological examination reveals a bitemporal upper quadrantic visual field defect.

a What is the likely diagnosis?

b Suggest two radiological and three endocrine investigations that should be done.

242

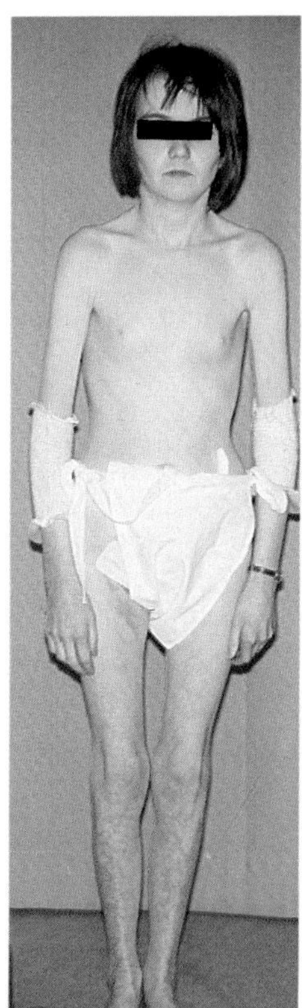

243

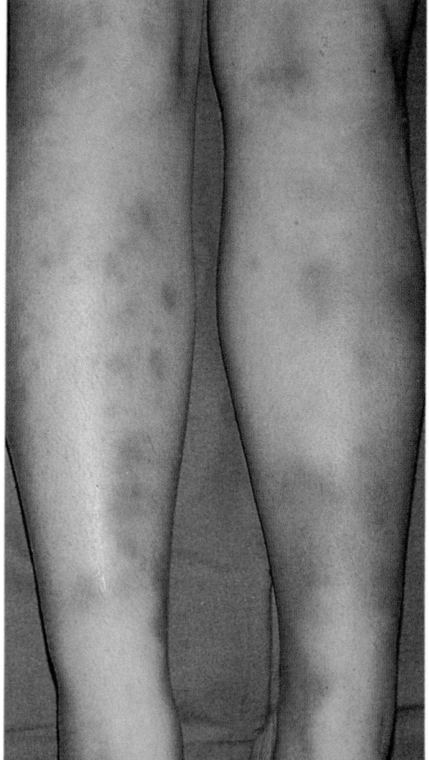

243

This twenty-three year old woman presented with a short history of pain and swelling in one knee, fever, and tender lumps over her shins and forearms.

a What are these lesions on her shins?

b Suggest three causes of her illness.

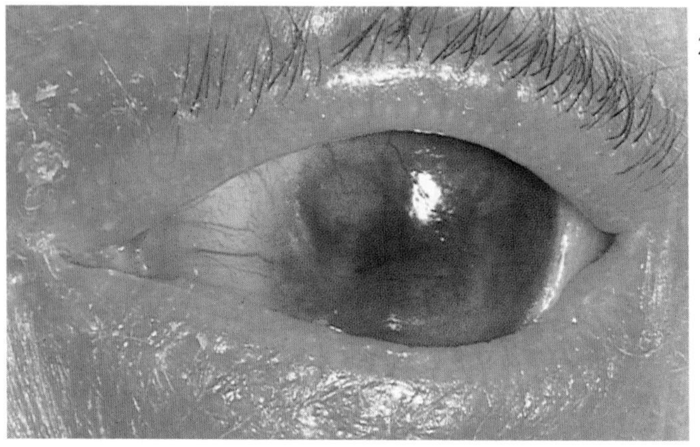

244

244 and 245 This teenage boy complains of pain and loss of vision, initially in the left eye alone, but affecting the right eye a few months later. The abdominal x-ray is that of his mother.

a What is the cause of his visual loss?
b What principal abnormality is seen on the x-ray?
c What is the underlying diagnosis?

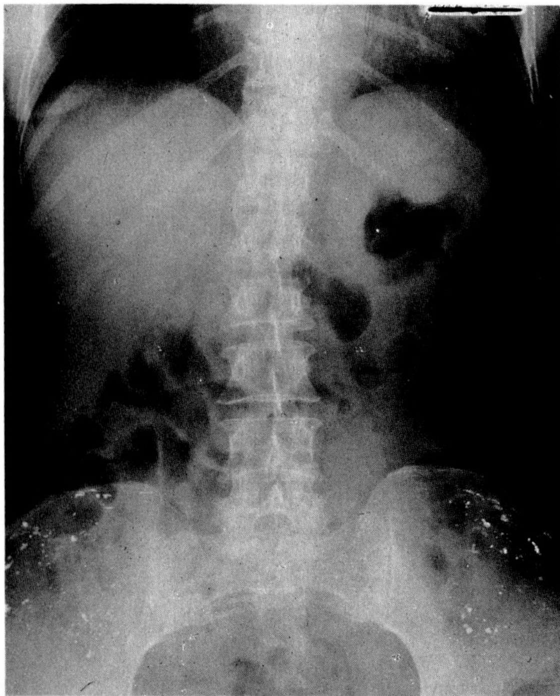

245

246
This patient is of Central African origin.

a What abnormality is seen in the ocular fundus?
b What are the two most common infective causes of such an appearance?

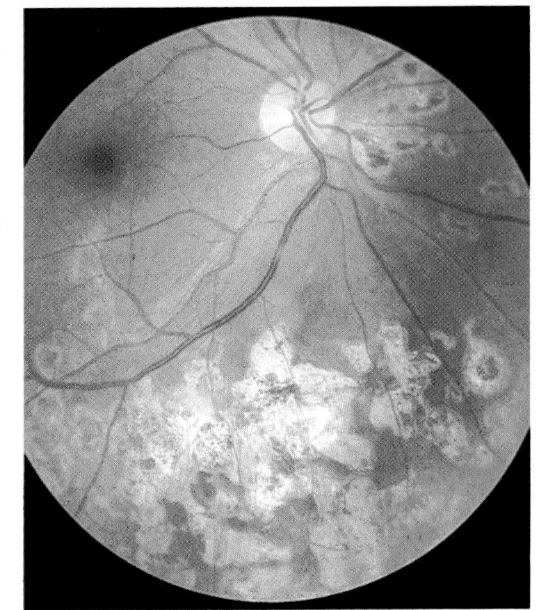

246

247
This patient has scabies.

a Which variety of this condition gives rise to the appearance seen in this finger web?
b What is the causative agent?
c List three conditions which may predispose to this variety.

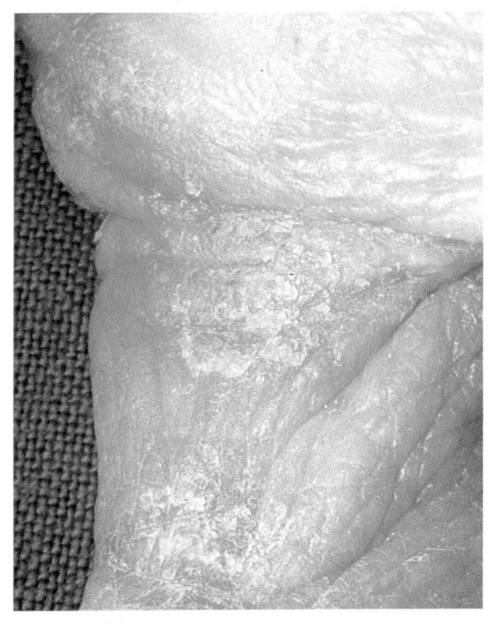

247

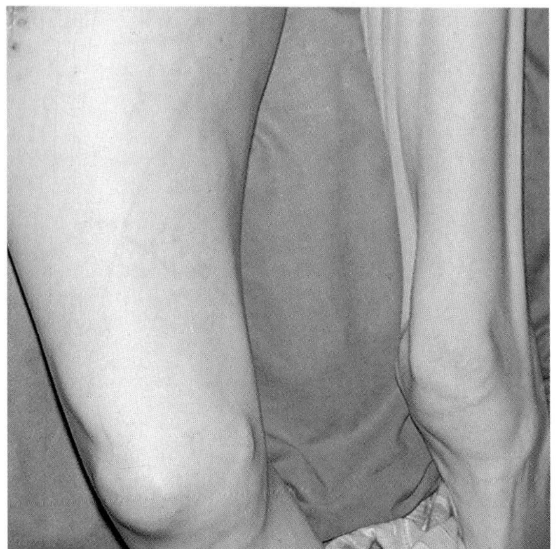

248

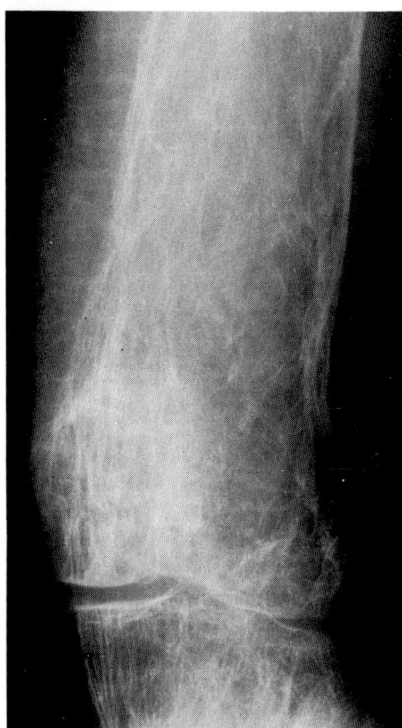

249

248 and 249 This elderly male patient suffers from a chronic bony disorder. Recently he has complained of pain in the right thigh.

a List four physical abnormalities seen in the legs.
b What radiological abnormalities are visible?
c What is the underlying disorder?
d What is the cause of his pain?

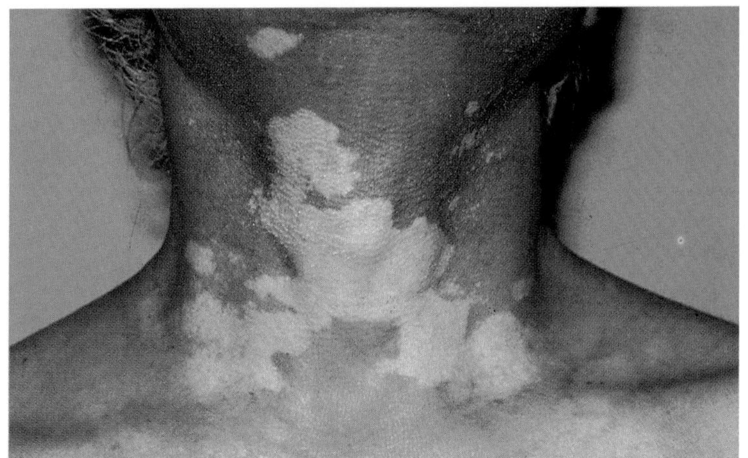

250

250

a What skin lesion is shown in this Asian patient?

b What endocrinopathies are associated with this skin condition?

251

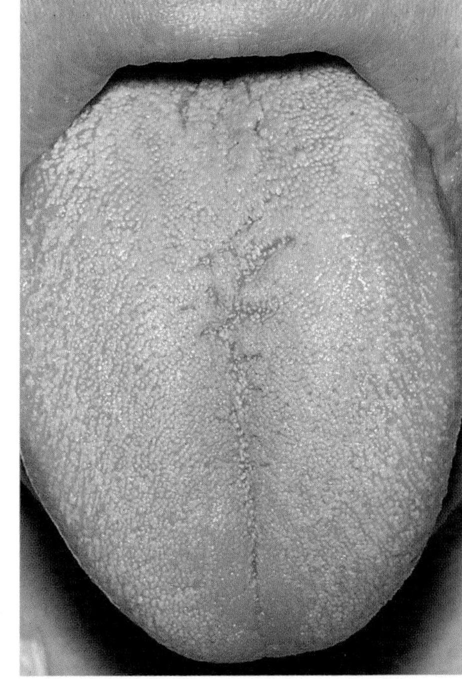

251

This patient is hypertensive.

a What abnormality is seen here?

b What unusual underlying cause for his hypertension does this suggest?

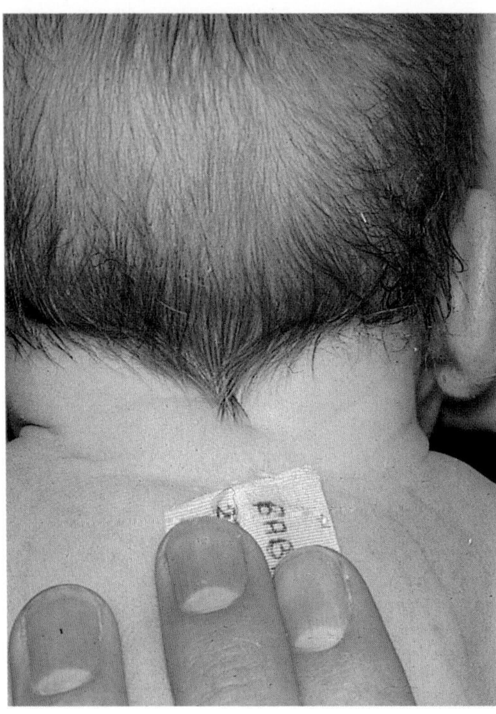

252

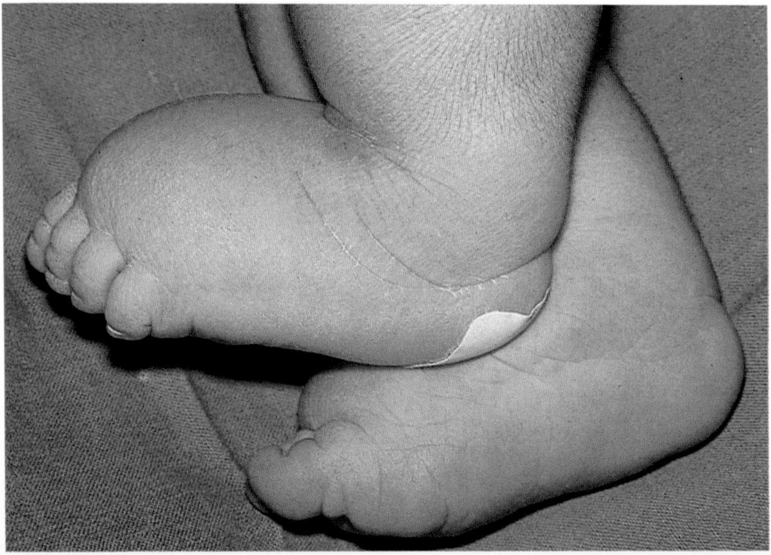

253

252 and 253
Buccal smear from this phenotypically female child is chromatin-negative.

a What abnormalities are seen in
   i) neck?
   ii) feet?

b What is the likely diagnosis?

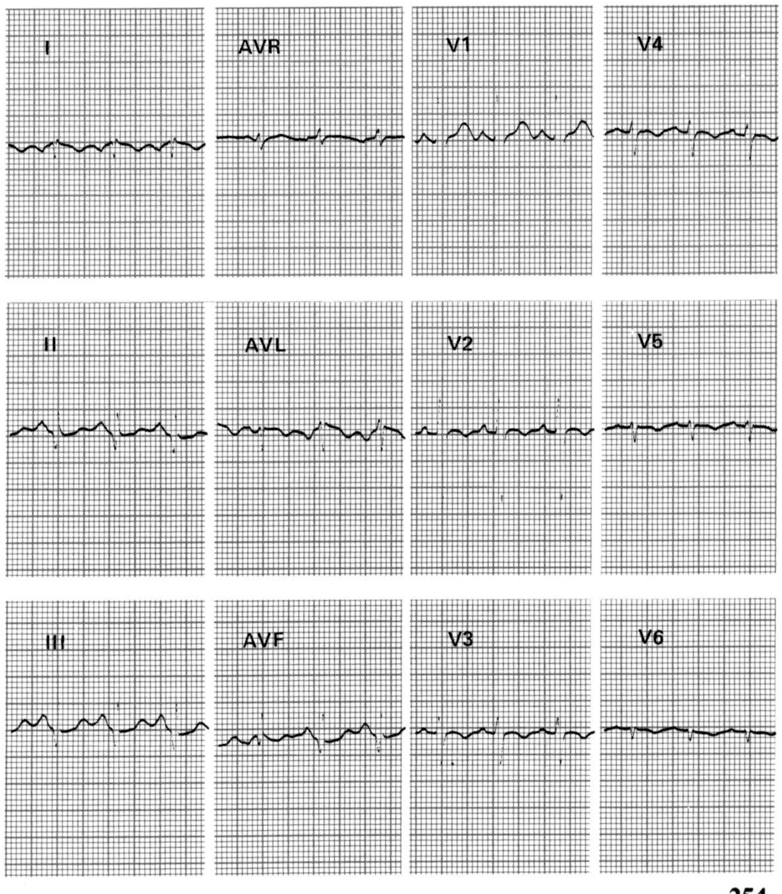

254

254 This woman with a past history of bronchiectasis was admitted with a further exacerbation. The ECG technician was chastised by the resident medical officer for transposing the limb leads of the ECG.

a Was the resident correct?
b Which diagnosis should be considered?
c What other symptoms may she have?

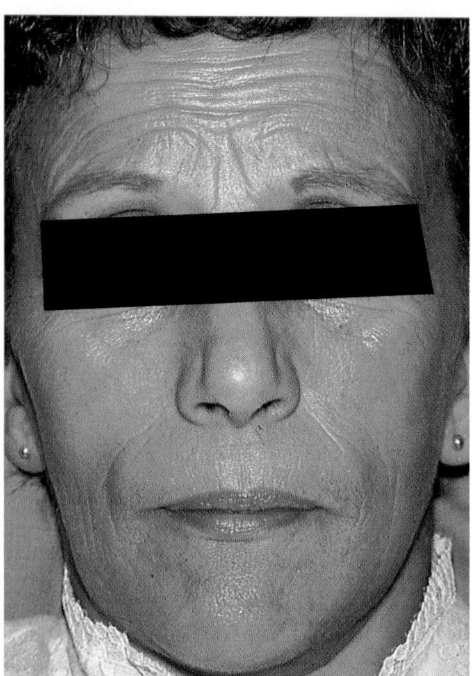

255

255

This woman has 'bronze diabetes'.

a What is unusual about the diagnosis in this patient?
b What is the cause of the pigmentation?
c What is the mode of inheritance of this disease?
d What is the effect of venesection on
   i) diabetic control?
   ii) cardiac failure?
   iii) risk of hepatoma?

256

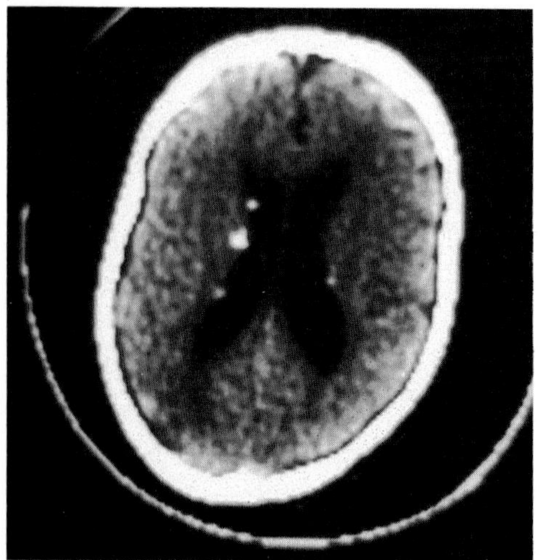

256

This person has epilepsy.

a What abnormality is present in this cerebral CT scan?
b What is the diagnosis?
c What cardiac abnormality is associated with this condition?

257

This person's blood film shows acanthocytosis.

a What abnormality is demonstrated?

b What is the association between these conditions?

c What neurological symptoms may occur?

d What therapy may be helpful in their prevention?

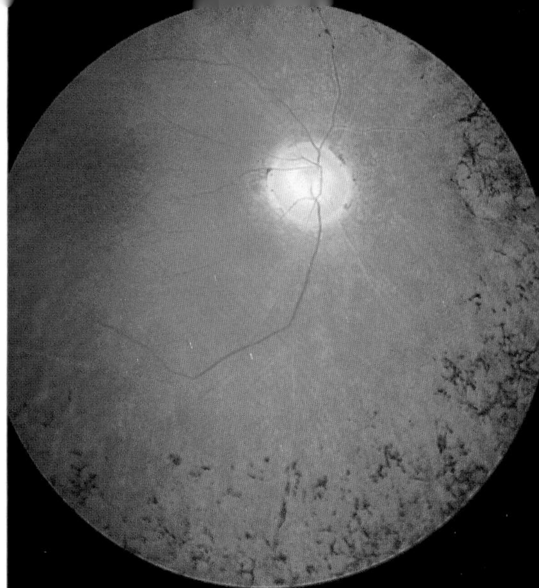

257

258

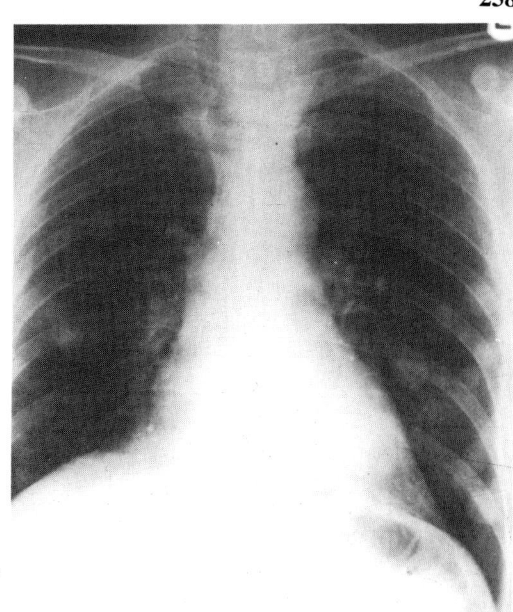

258

a What two abnormalities are seen on this chest x-ray?

b What is the most likely diagnosis?

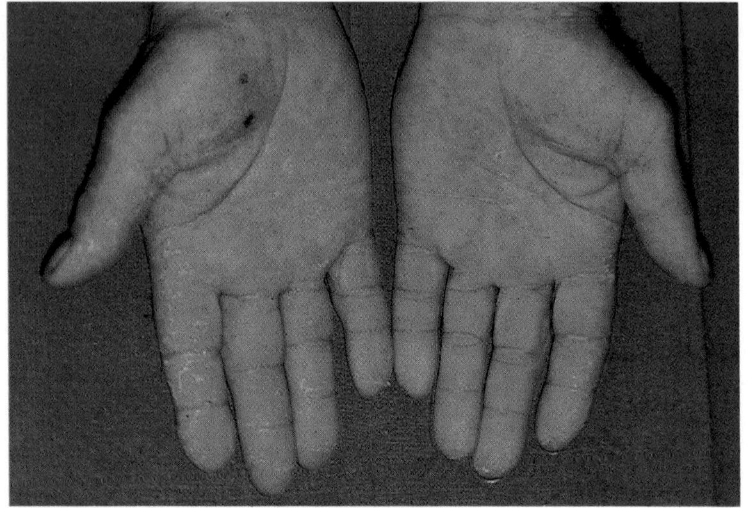

259

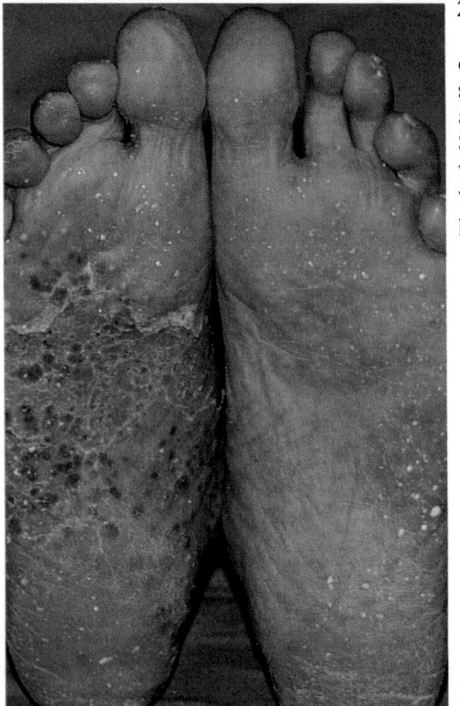

260

259 and 260

This patient complains of pain and swelling of his knee joints and of painful red eyes. Suggest two diagnoses which link his symptoms with the appearance of his palms and soles.

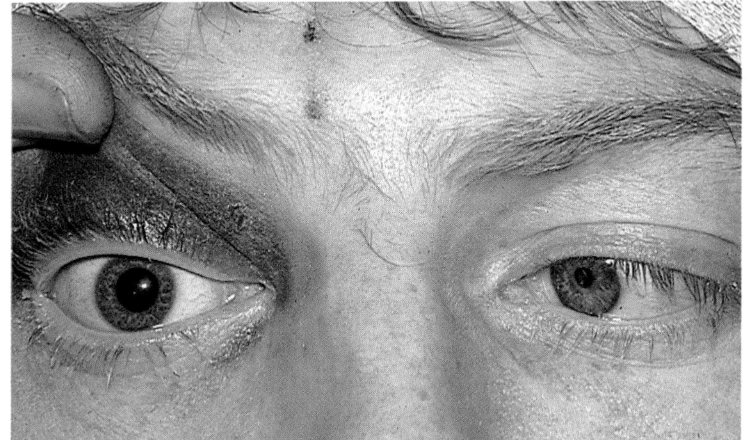

261

261 This patient is attempting to look down and to his right.
a What neurological abnormalities are demonstrated?
b From his appearance, suggest three possible causes.

262

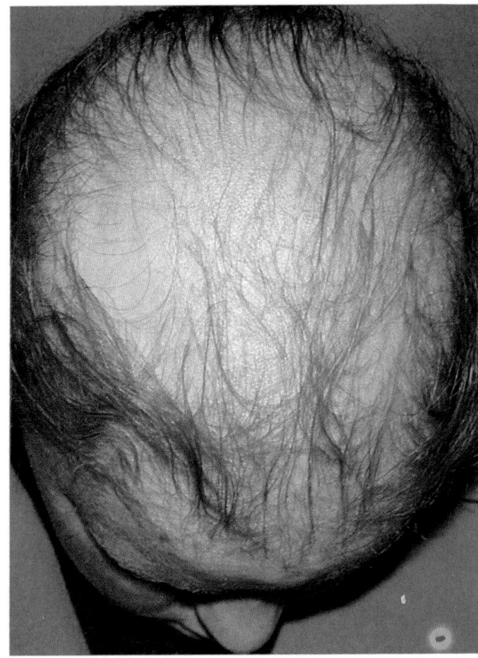

262
Which congenital abnormality is most typically associated with this appearance in a young patient?

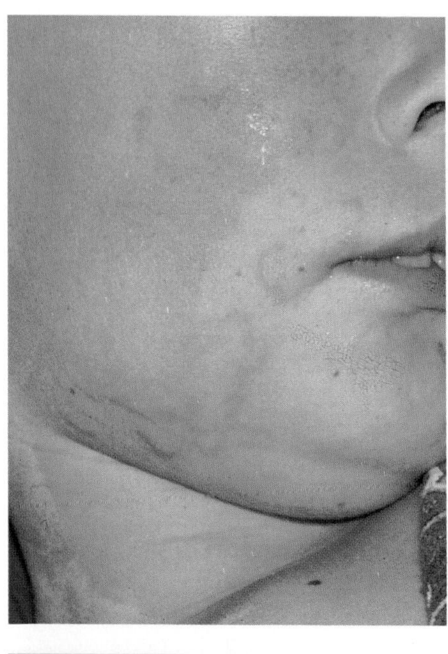

263

263

What is the cause of this child's recently diagnosed apical diastolic murmur?

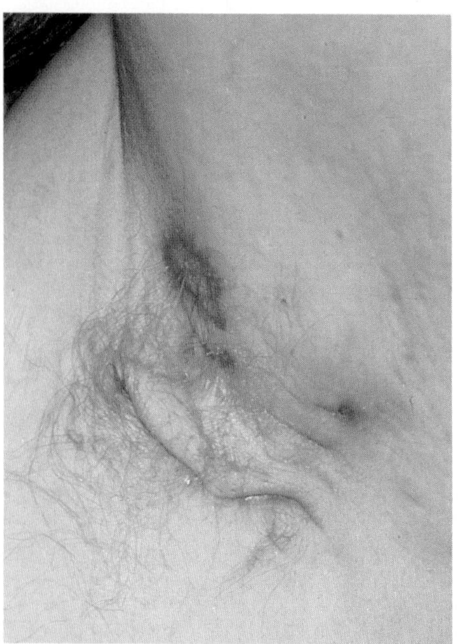

264

264

a What is the most likely cause of the abnormality seen in this twenty-six year old female patient's axilla?

b Which infective agent is usually responsible?

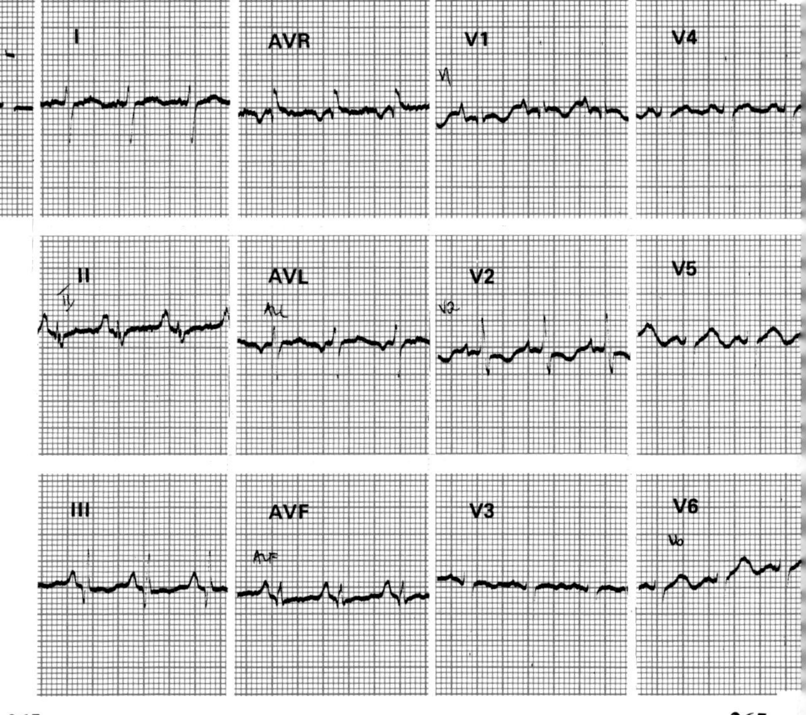

265 **265**

This thirty-eight year old woman suffers from bronchiectasis following an attack of measles in childhood.

a What are the ECG abnormalities?

b What condition has developed?

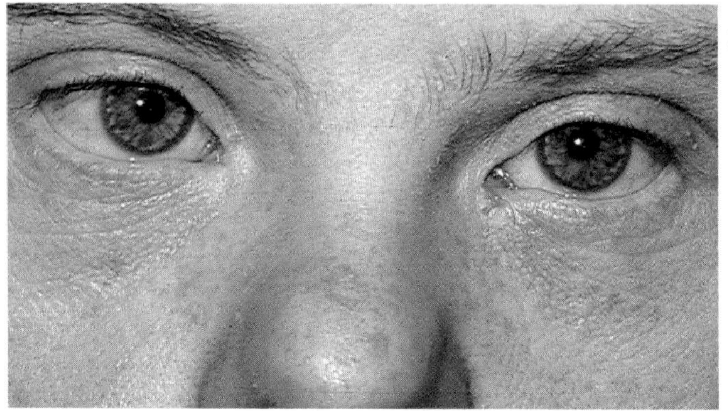

266

266
This patient has Down's syndrome. His mother was twenty-two years old when he was born.

a List two possible chromosomal abnormalities consistent with this syndrome.
b List the possible underlying defective genetic mechanisms in order of likelihood.

267
a What abnormality is seen in this lateral skull x-ray?
b Of what condition is this appearance characteristic?
c List four other conditions which may give rise to a similar appearance in this area.

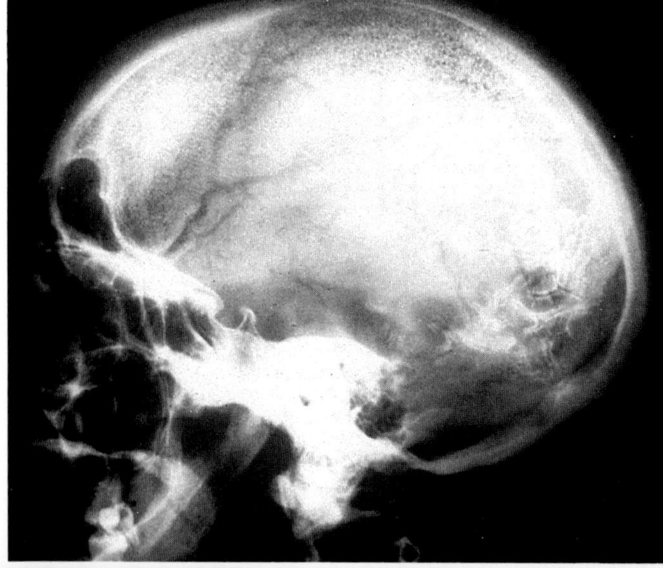

267

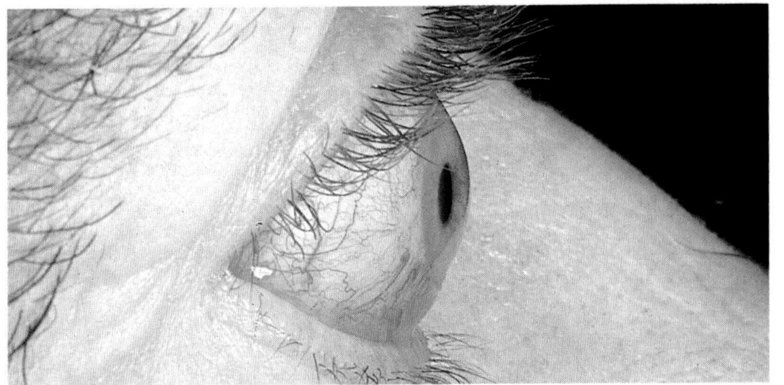

268

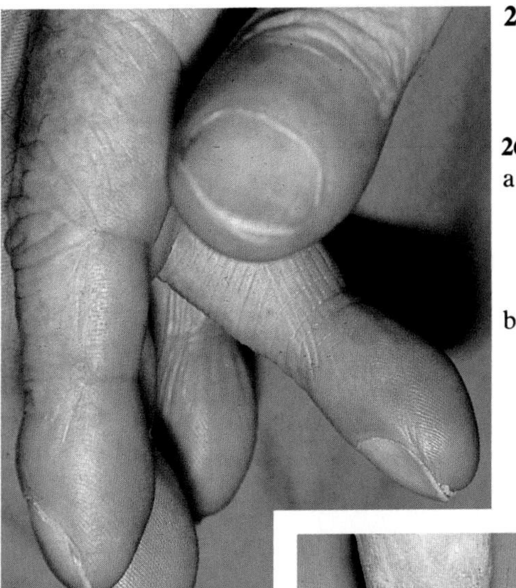

269

268, 269 and 270

a What abnormalities are seen in these patients'
  i) eye?
  ii) hands?
  iii) legs?

b Which endocrine disorder is typified by this triad?

270

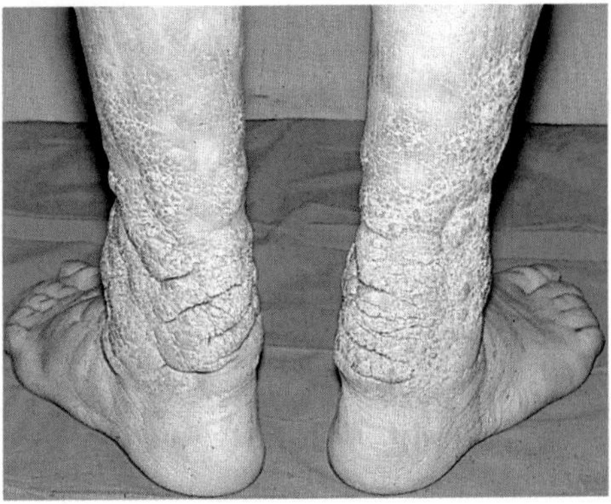

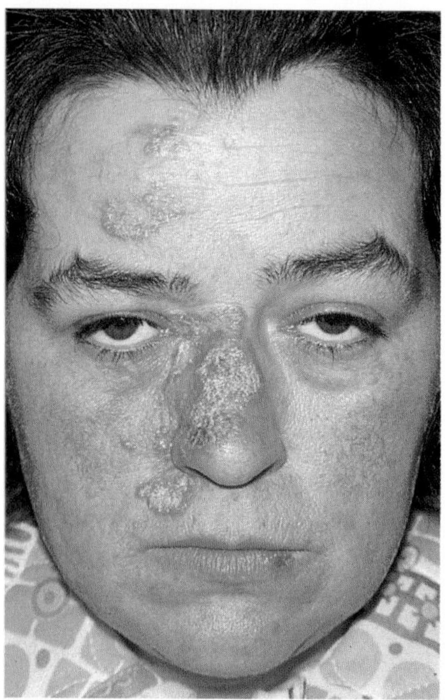

271

a What is this condition?
b What are the important clinical dermatological features?
c What is the incidence of systemic lupus erythematosus in this disease?

271

272 a What is the cause of the abnormal appearance of this child's eye?
b What is its aetiology?
c At which other sites may it be found in the orbit?

272

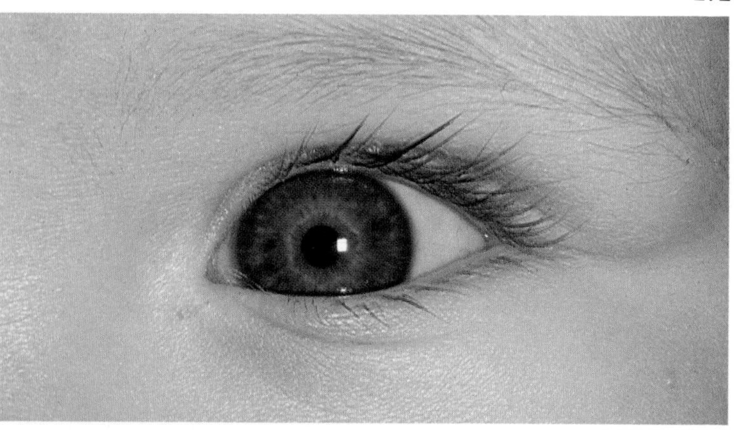

273

This fifty year old man sustained an anterior myocardial infarction. Four days after admission he suddenly became breathless, hypotensive, and peripherally cyanosed. A loud pansystolic murmur was noted.

a What is the radiological diagnosis?
b What is the likely cause of his deterioration?

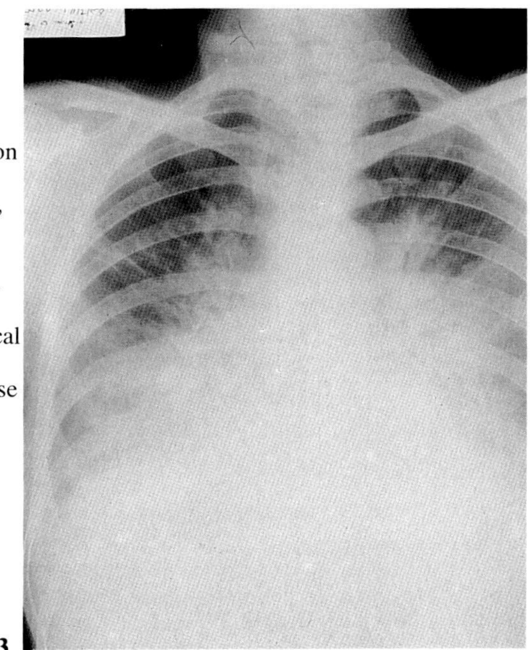

273

274 This man complained of pain on swallowing and pain in his right ear.

a Describe the abnormality present?
b What is the likely diagnosis?
c What factors are involved in its aetiology?

274

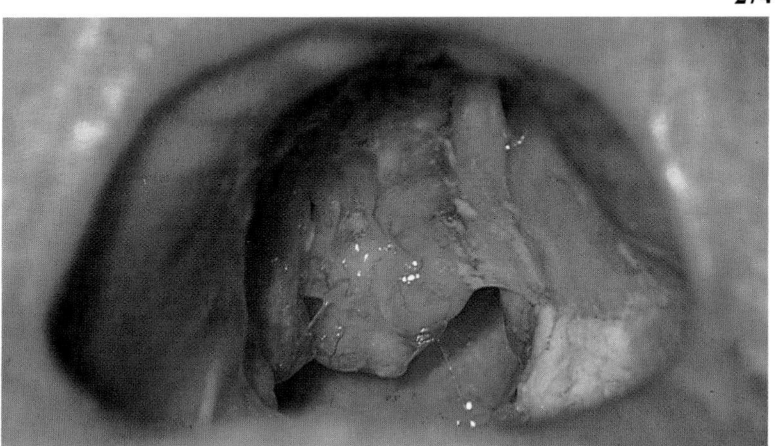

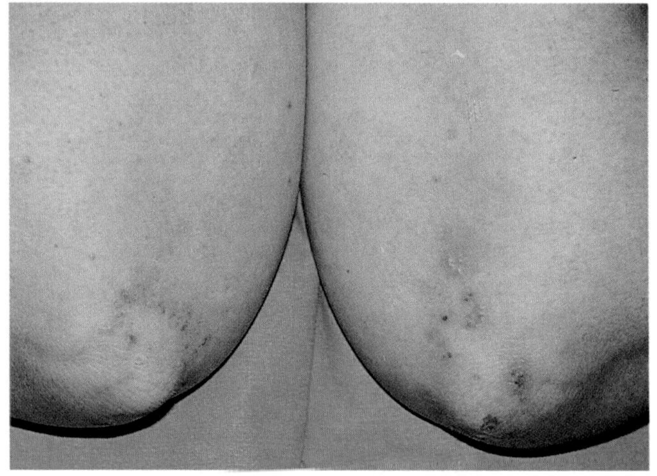

276

275, 276, 277 and 278 These four patients suffer from recurrent bullous eruptions.

Patient 1

complains of an intensely pruritic eruption on his elbows (as shown), knees and buttocks. Topical corticosteroid applications have failed to alleviate the pruritus.

Patient 2

is seventy-five years old. She suffers from recurrent episodes of blistering of arms, legs and trunk. The blisters are tense, do not rupture easily, and heal without scarring.

275

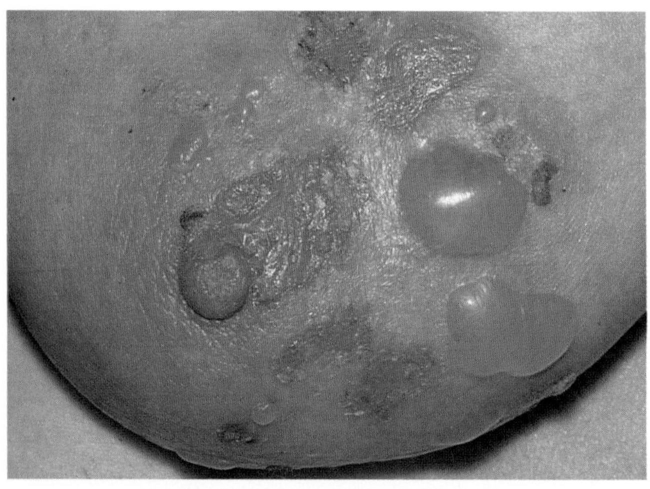

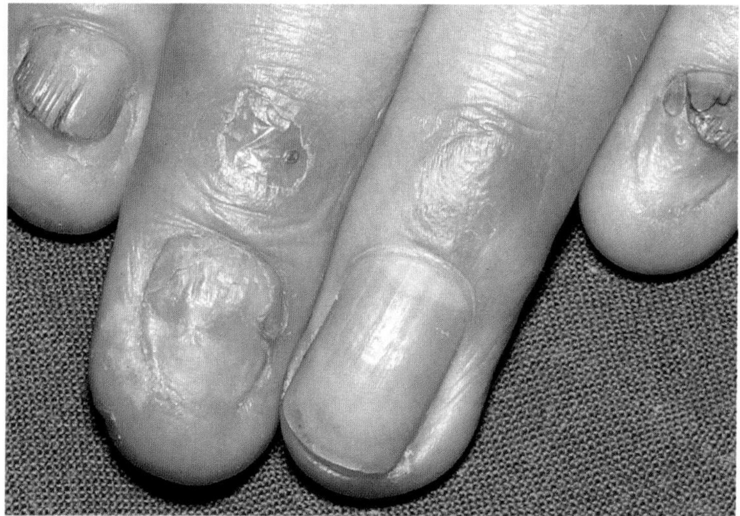

277

278

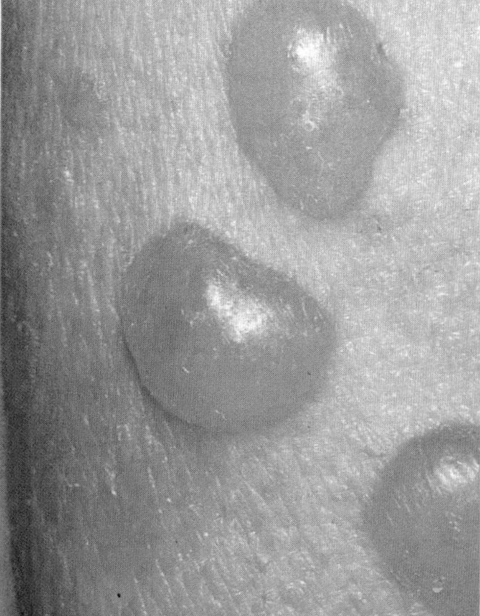

Patient 3
has a strong family history of blistering disease. From early childhood, minor trauma has caused blistering. The blisters heal with scarring as shown.

Patient 4
is fifty-two years old. Several months ago she complained of recurrent painful lesions of the buccal mucosa. The blisters seen here are confined to the left arm. They are easily broken, leaving painful, raw areas beneath.

Give the most likely diagnosis in each case.

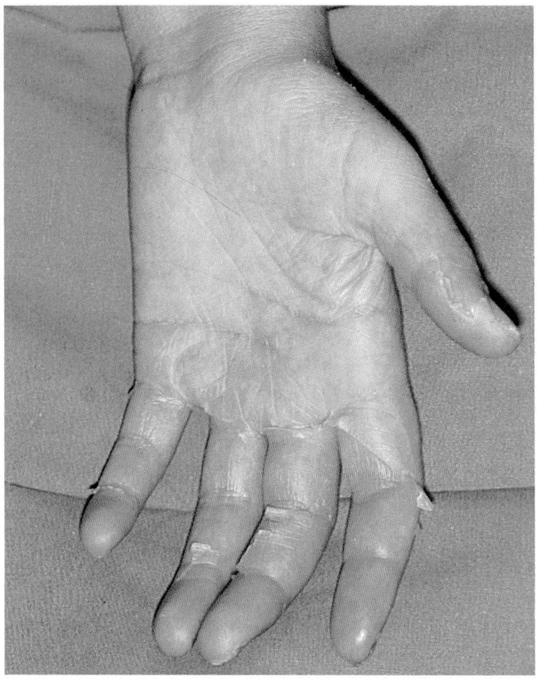

279

279 and 280 These conditions have an aetiological link.

a What are the conditions?
b What is the link?
c What accounts for the differing clinical presentation?

280

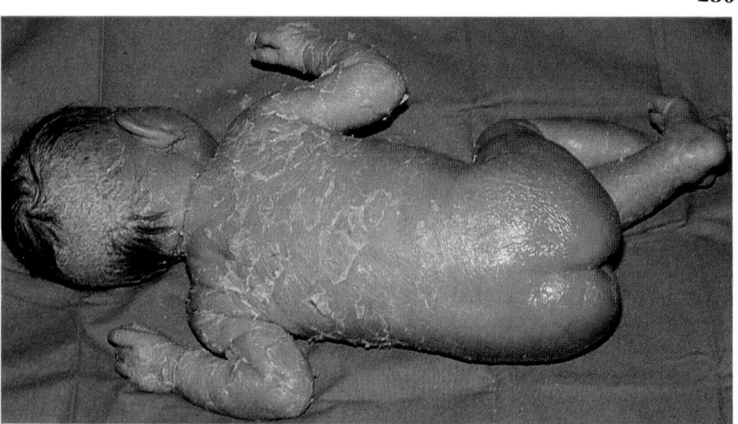

281

This patient is attempting to smile.

a What is the diagnosis?
b By which investigation is this most easily established?
c What other investigations are useful?

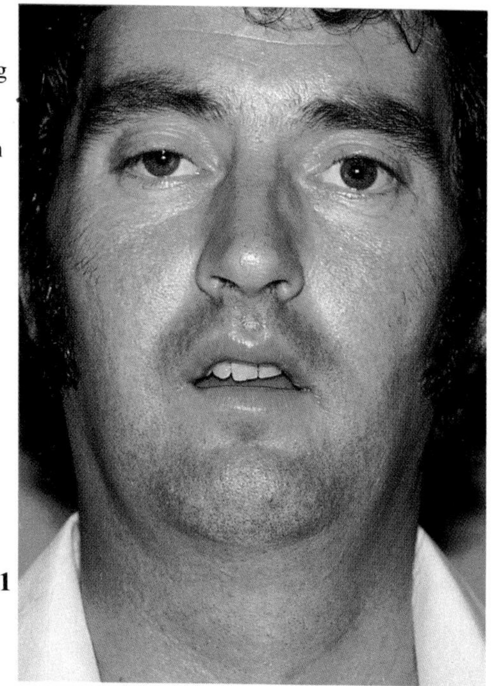

281

282

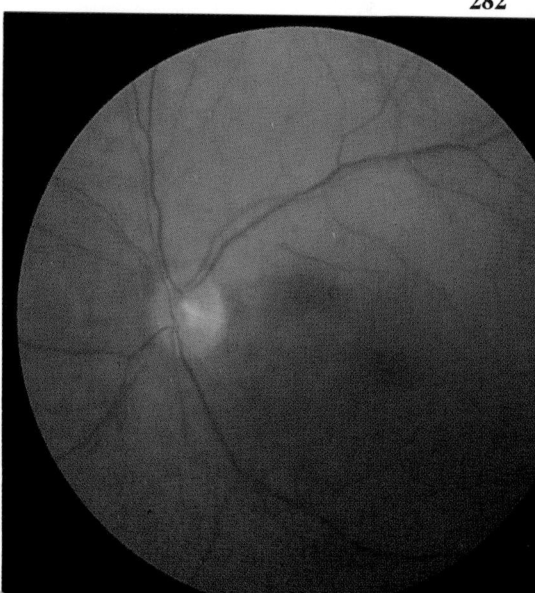

282

This patient has a recent history of pain in the tongue and jaw on chewing. Twelve hours ago she suddenly became blind in this eye.

a List three abnormalities visible in the optic fundus.
b What is the diagnosis?
c Would you expect the indirect light reflex in this eye to be normal?
d What underlying diagnosis must be considered?

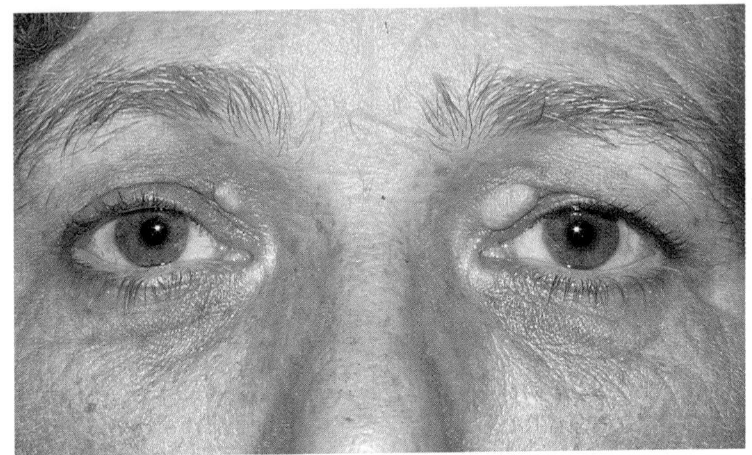

283

283 and 284 This thirty-six year old woman has a strong family history of ischaemic heart disease.

a What abnormality is seen adjacent to her eyelids?

b What substance is responsible for the yellow discolouration of her hands?

c Suggest five conditions which may be associated with both abnormalities.

284

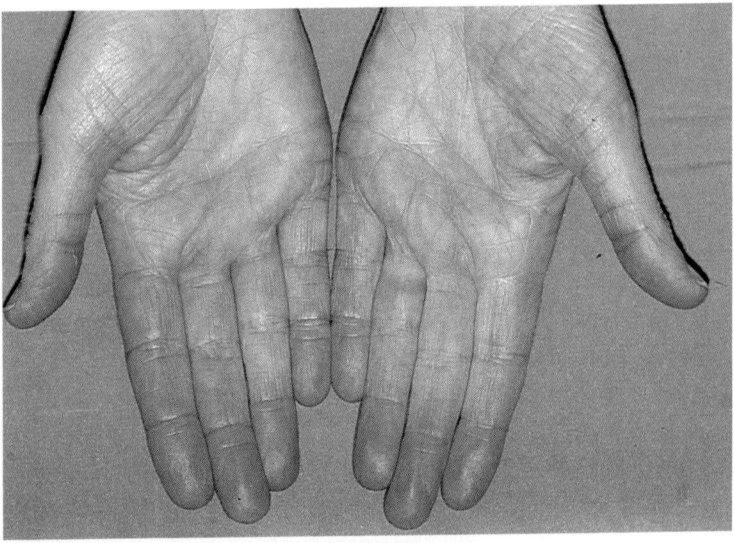

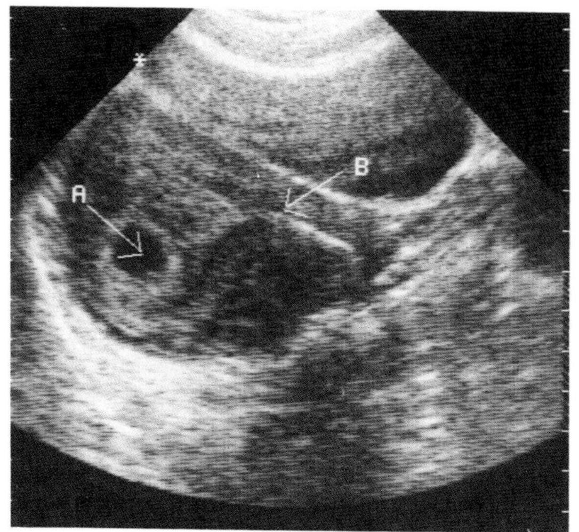

285

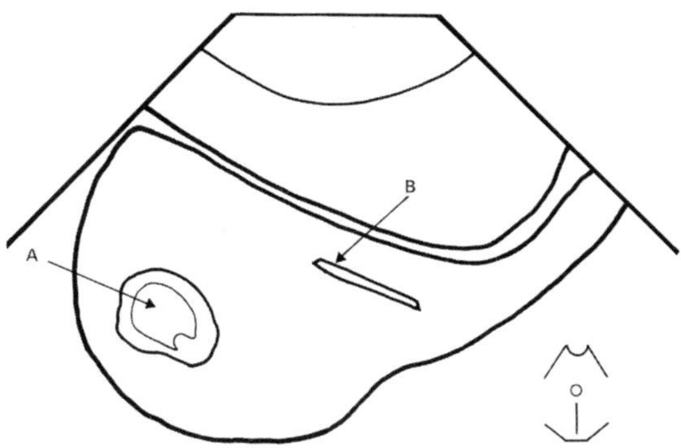

285 This nineteen year old girl presented with back pain in the lower lumbar area. A pelvic mass was found on examination and a diagnosis of ovarian cyst was made.

a Does this sagittal ultrasonic pelvic scan confirm this diagnosis?
b Name the features labelled 'A' and 'B'.

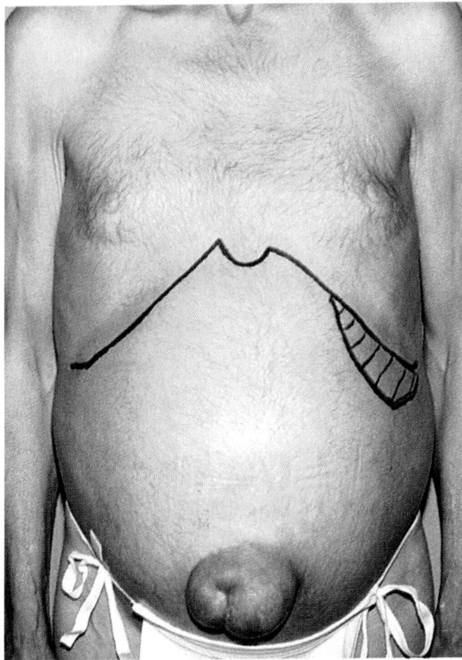

286

286

This patient has ascites.

a In addition to splenomegaly (delineated in pen) which two other principal abnormalities are visible?

b What is, approximately, the smallest amount of ascitic fluid which can be detected clinically? By which unusual test may this be detected?

287

This patient works in a glue factory. The lesion seen on her left cheek began as a small scratch a week ago. Over the past four days the lesion has enlarged rapidly. She now complains of headache and malaise. Her temperature is 38°C and pulse rate 90/minute.

a What other facial abnormality is seen?

287

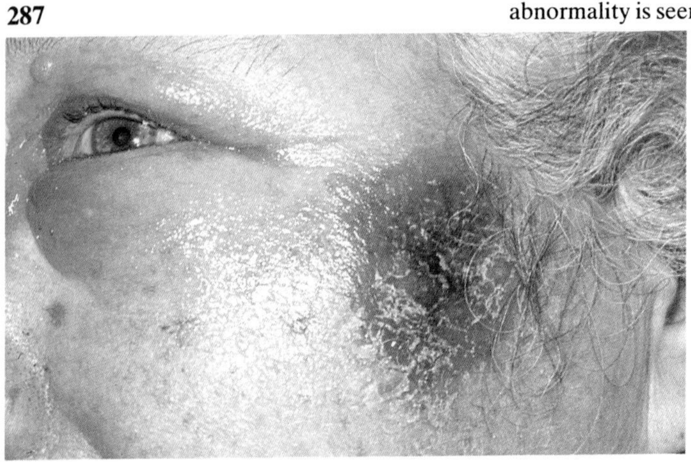

b Of which unusual infection is this appearance typical?
c What other conditions may give rise to a similar appearance?
d Is specific treatment necessary?

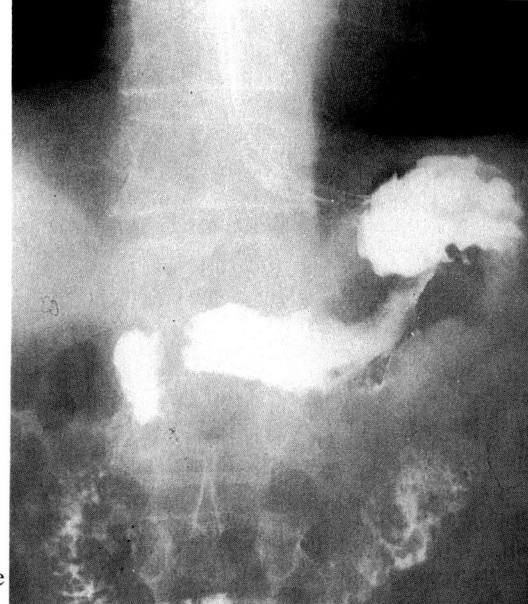

288

288
This fifty year old male patient complains of weight loss and fullness after meals.
a What abnormality is seen on barium meal?
b What descriptive name is given to this lesion?

289

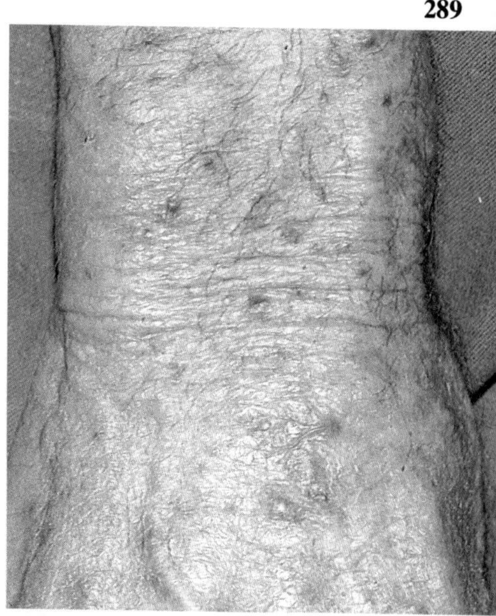

289
This patient has an iron deficiency anaemia. Faecal occult blood analysis is consistently positive. Gastroscopy, sigmoidoscopy and barium series have demonstrated no abnormalities.
a What unusual diagnosis is suggested by the appearance of the skin of his forearm?
b What is the source of blood loss in this condition?
c In which other sites may similar lesions occur?

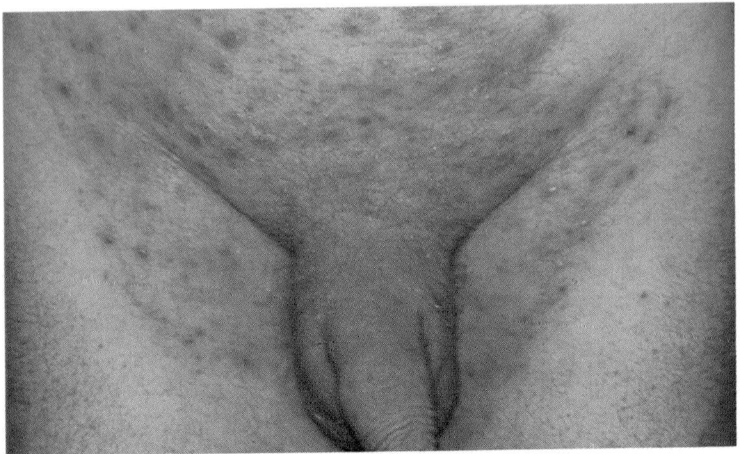

290

291

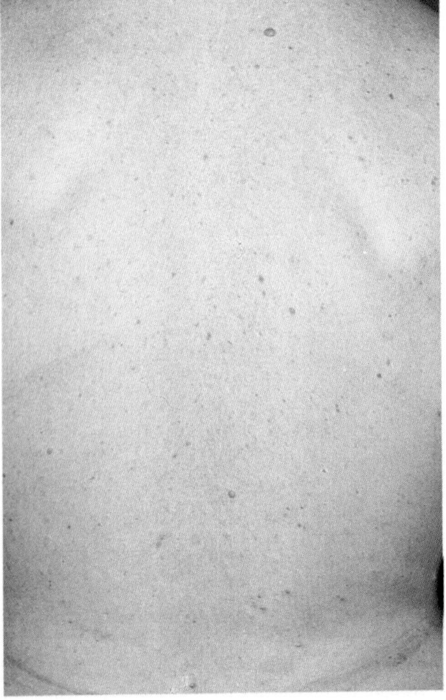

290

This man's itchy rash flared up when he applied a topical steroid cream.

a What is the likely underlying aetiology?

b What therapy should he have been prescribed?

291

This thirty-three year old woman presented with left sensorineural deafness and tinnitus of three month's duration. Examination revealed an absent left corneal reflex.

a What two skin abnormalities are seen?

b What is the underlying disorder?

c What is the cause of her deafness?

292 This boy with choreoathetosis and a tendency to self mutilation has had several episodes of gout.

a What is the name of this condition?
b How is it inherited?
c Which enzyme is lacking?

293 This obese female patient has been admitted following a haematemesis.

a What name is given to the venous abnormality seen in relation to her umbilicus?
b What underlying haemodynamic disturbance does this imply?
Which three causes for her haematemesis should be considered?

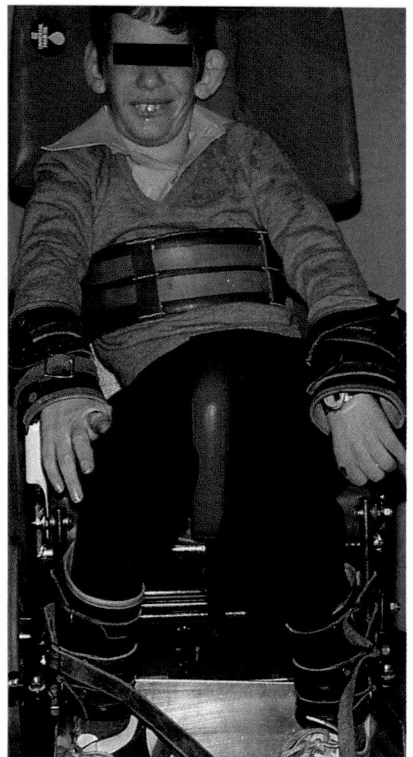

292

293

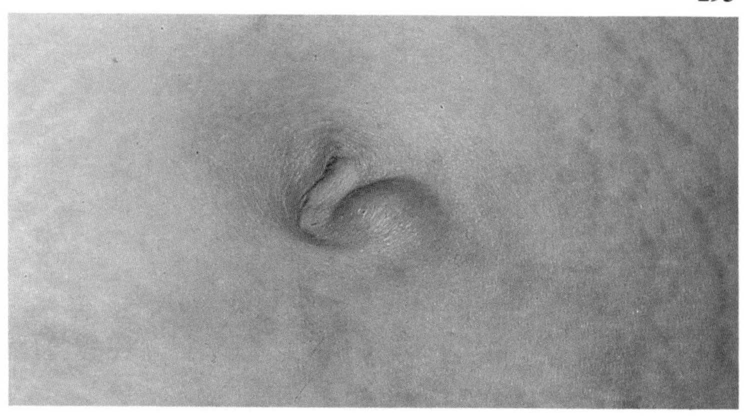

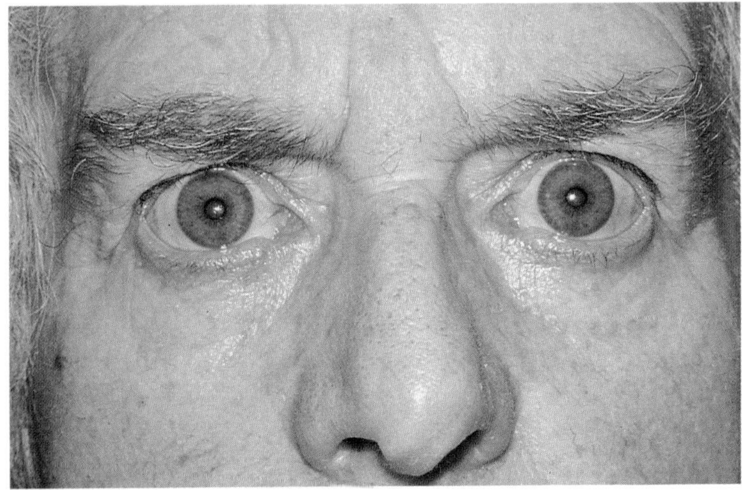

294

294 and 295

a What physical sign is being demonstrated here?
b What is the significance of a positive test?

295

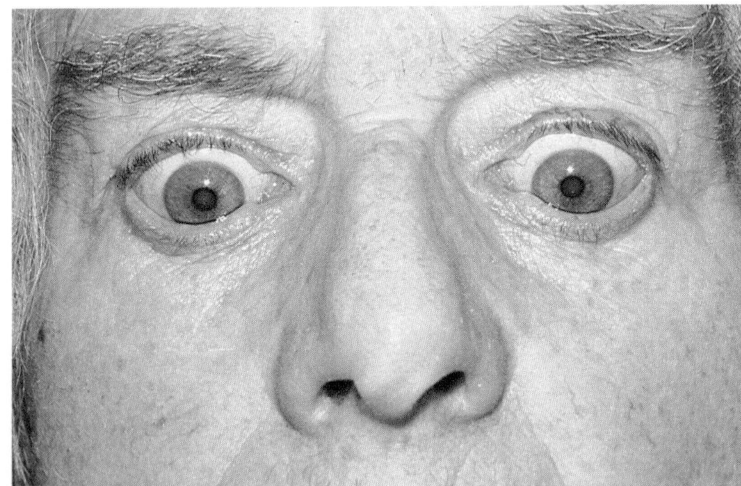

296

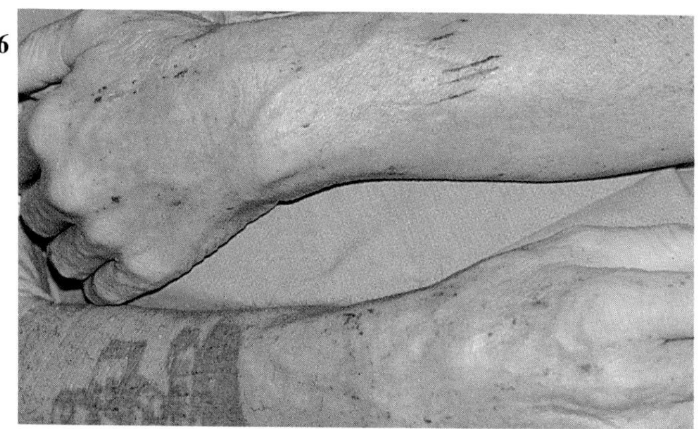

296 and 297

This patient has been admitted to your unit moribund and unable to give a history. He is hypotensive and clinically dehydrated, tachypnoeic with Kussmaul-type respiration. His previous case notes are not available, but you are able to locate his previous x-rays. Initial biochemical results are: Na 148 mmol/l, K 6.2 mmol/l, HCO_3 7 mmol/l, urea 42.0 mmol/l, creatinine 440 mol/l, plasma glucose 5.8 mmol/l.

a What abnormalties are seen
   i) in the hand x-rays?
   ii) on the skin of his arms?

b What important implication can be taken, with respect to his pre-existing renal function?

c What value, approximately, would you expect the urinary specific gravity to be?

297

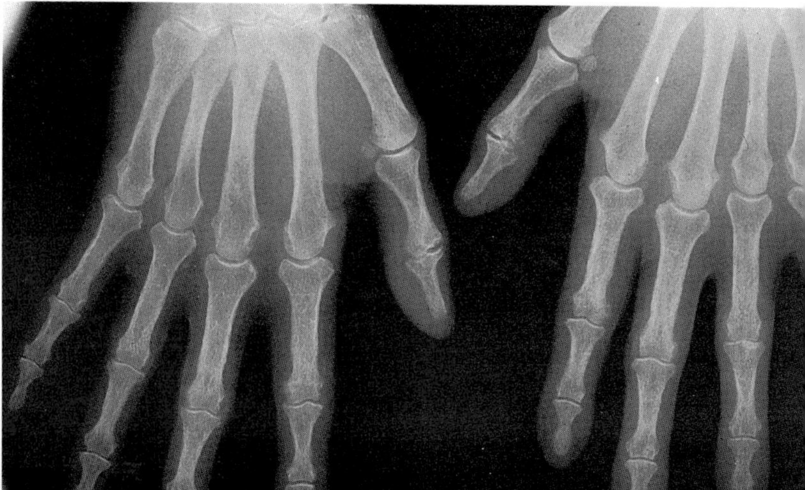

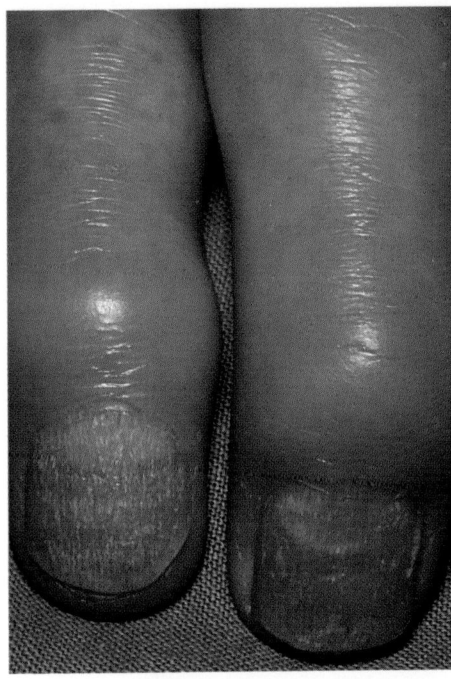

298 and 299 This patient complained of morning stiffness and pain in the small joints of the hand. A diagnosis of rheumatoid arthritis was made. After six months on a variety of nonsteroidal anti-inflammatory drugs he was given a 'second line' drug. Shortly afterwards he developed widespread erythroderma with pustulation.

a What was the true cause of his joint pains?
b Which 'second line' drug was he given?

298

299

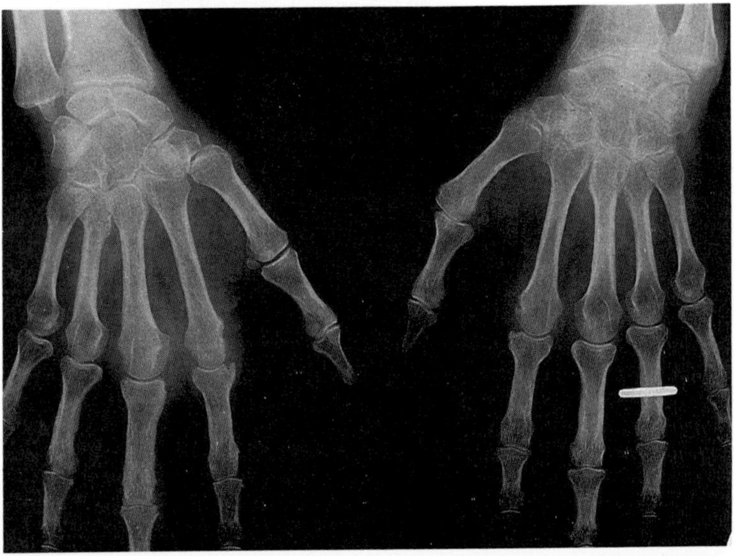

300

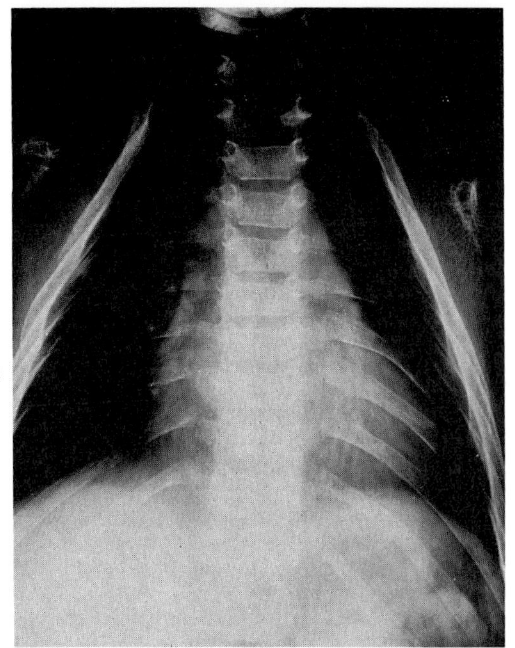

300

a What principal abnormality is seen on this chest radiograph?

b What is the diagnosis?

c In which two other sites would you expect to find radiological abnormalities in this condition?

301

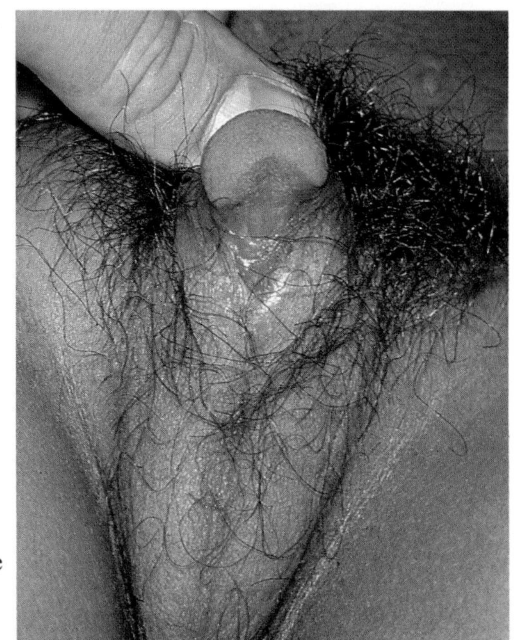

301

a What physical sign is demonstrated here?

b What is the significance of this finding?

302

302

This woman presented with a six month history of general ill-health, weight loss of two stones, and light headedness.

a What diagnosis does her appearance suggest?
b How should the diagnosis be confirmed?
c What abnormalities may a differential white cell count show?

303

a What is this appearance?
b In which diseases may it occur?

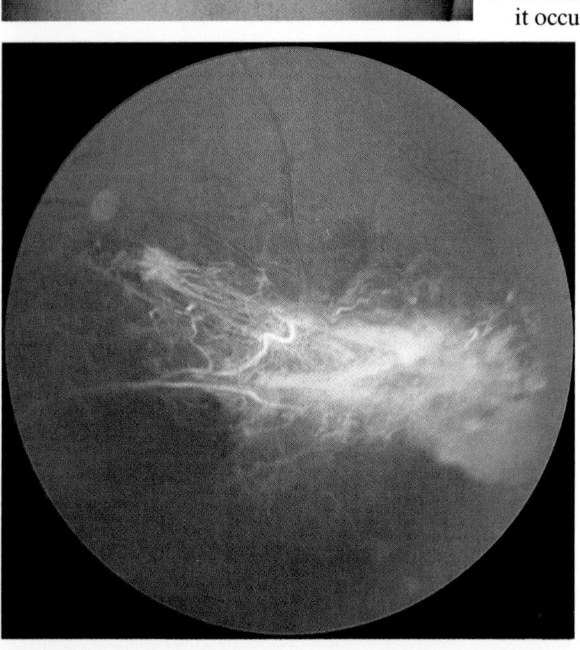

303

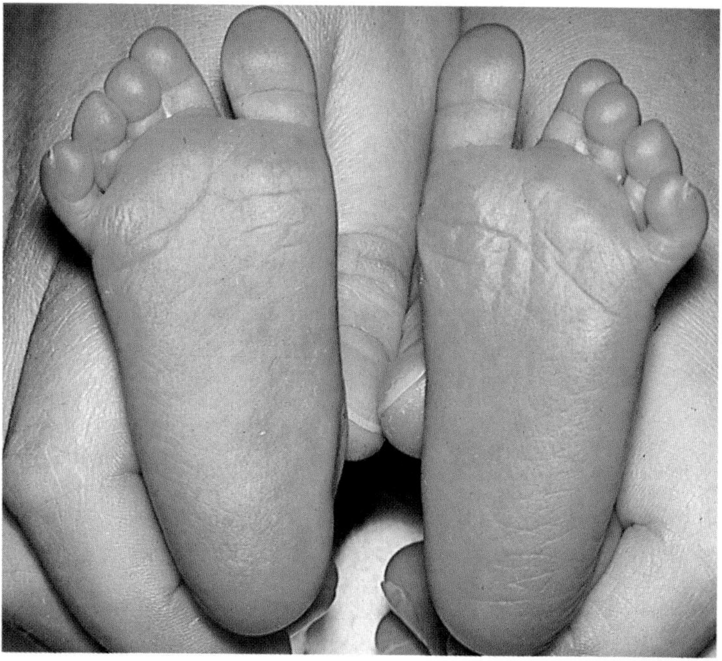

304 Is this a full term baby? **304**

305 a What is the cause of this appearance?
b What effect on function occurs?
c What iatrogenic factor may be involved? **305**

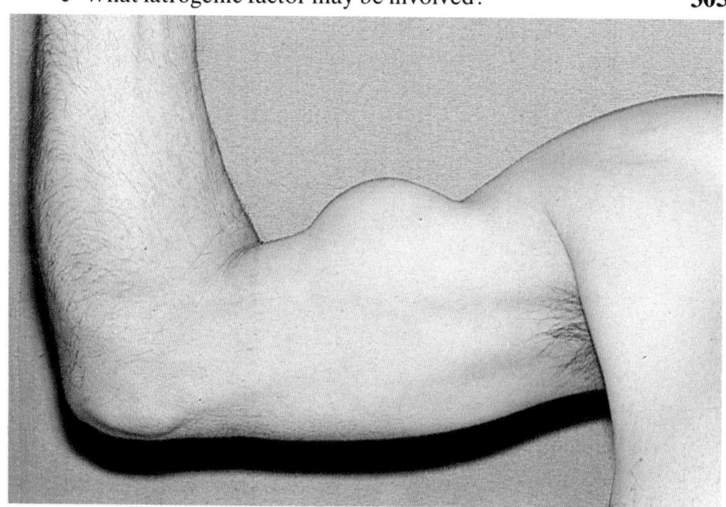

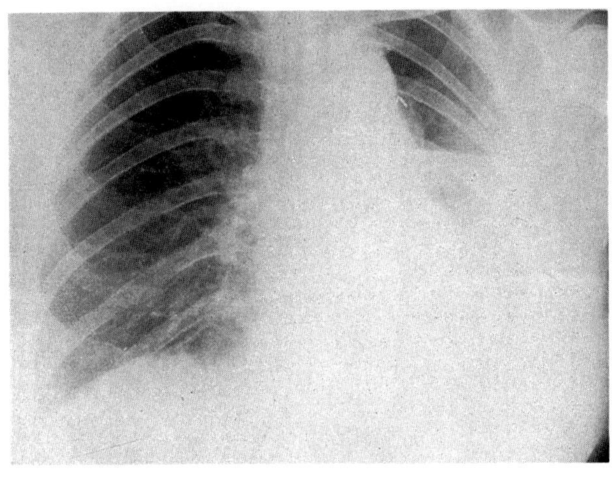

306

306 and 307 These x-rays were taken three years apart, the lower most recently.

a List four radiological abnormalities visible in the upper x-ray.

b What new abnormality has developed in the lower x-ray?

c What is the likely diagnosis?

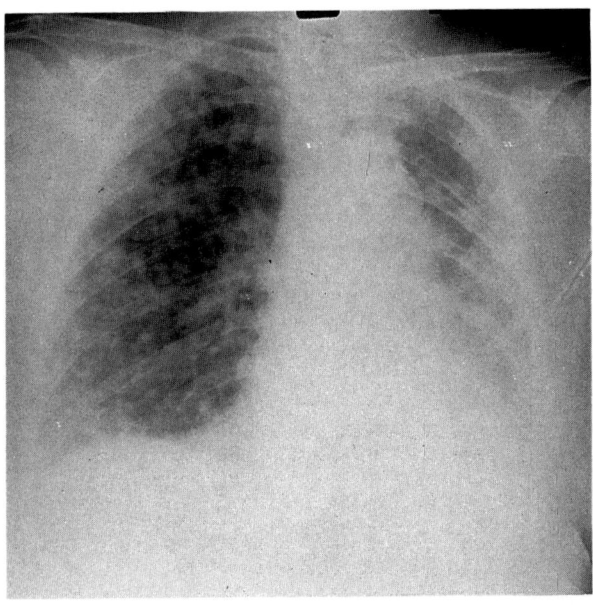

307

308

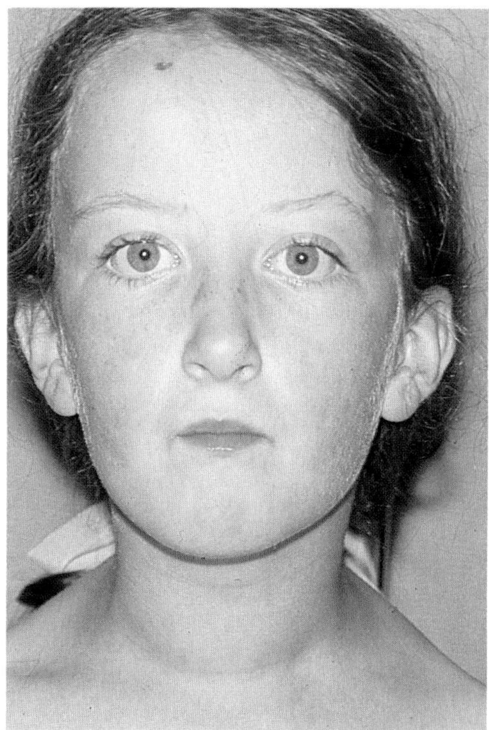

308
This girl is clinically mildly hyperthyroid. Her total serum thyroxine (T4) concentration is at the upper limit of normal at 148 nmol/l. She has received neither antithyroid nor ablative therapy. Suggest five possible reasons for the apparently low T4.

309
This seventy year old lady was admitted with acute abdominal pain radiating through to her back. The pain was accompanied by abdominal tenderness.
Name the structures labelled 1 to 5 on this CT scan of the lower abdomen (following intravenous injection of contrast medium).

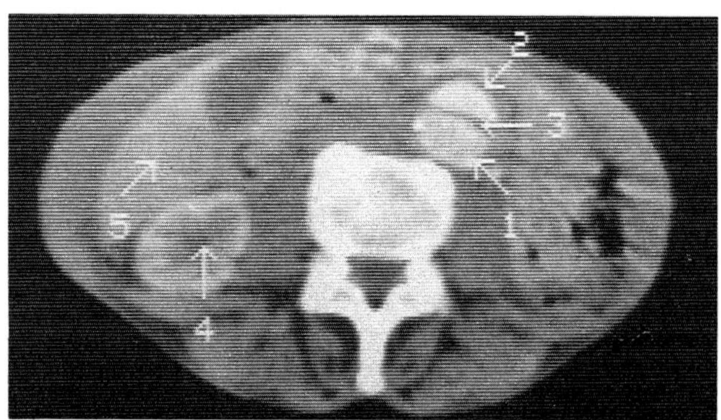

309

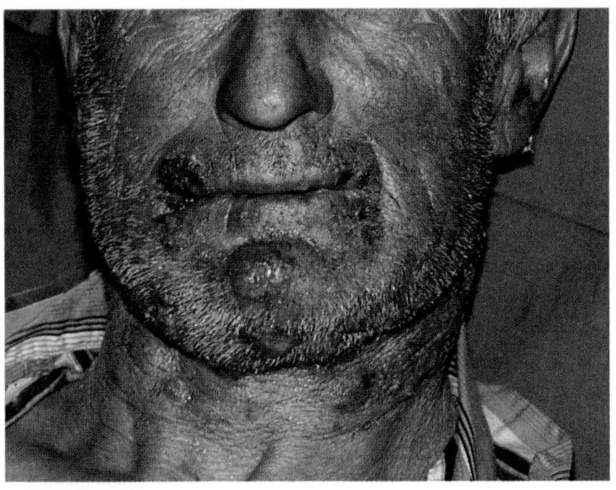

310

310 This farmer blamed his cows for his facial appearance.
a Is he correct?
b What is the diagnosis?
c What treatment is indicated?

311 Name four organisms which may cause this appearance.

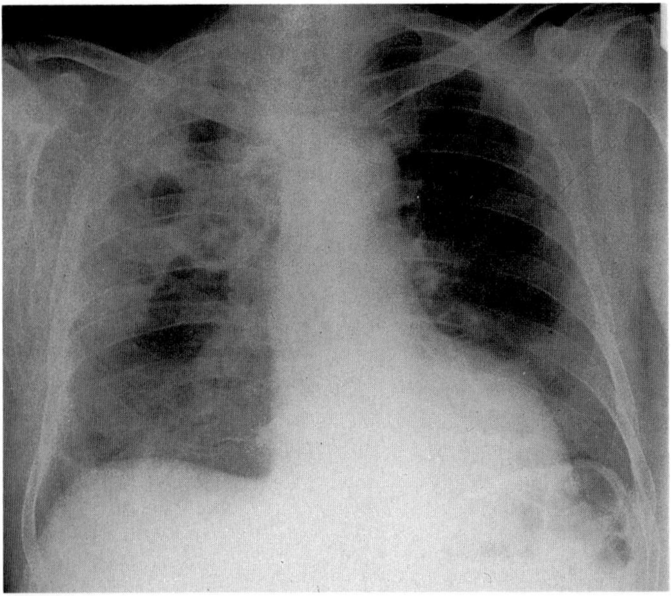

311

312

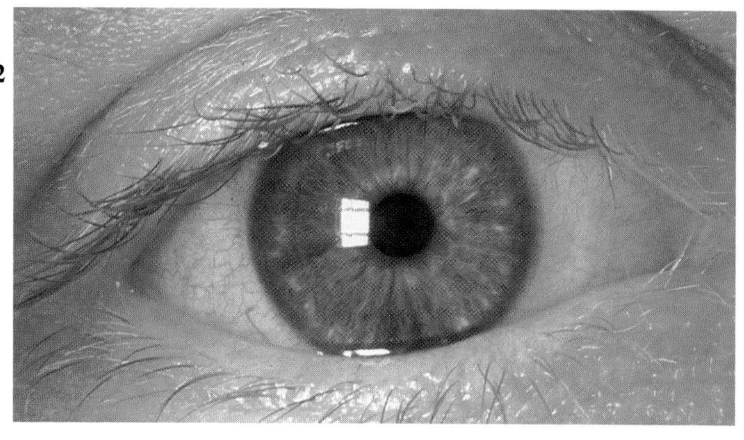

312
This patient is a fish-filleter. She developed severe headache and myalgia, followed by sore eyes. On admission, she was jaundiced, had calf pain and microscopic haematuria.
a What is the likely diagnosis?
b Is her occupation relevant?
c What is the major vector of the disease?

313
This child developed an itchy papule on the dorsum of his hand which has continued to spread.
a What is the diagnosis?
b Which agent is usually responsible?

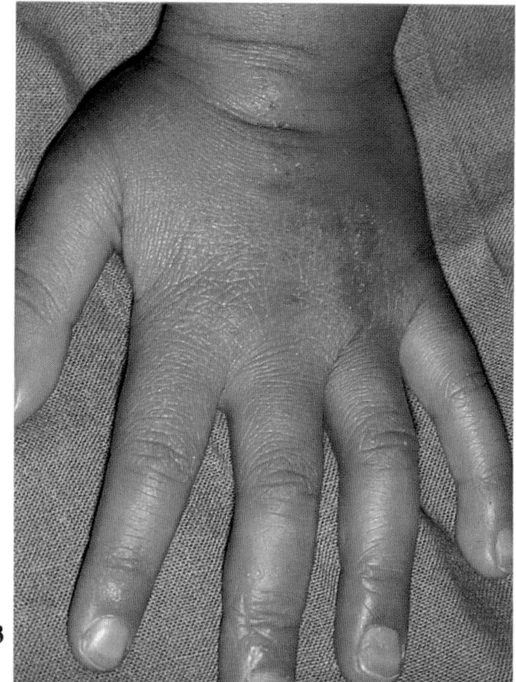

313

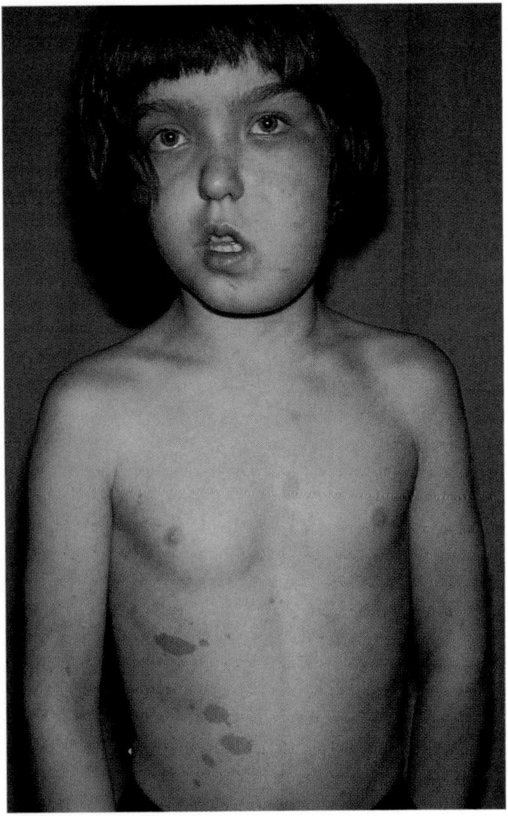

314
This child's facial nerve palsy has an unusual underlying cause. Suggest what this cause may be.

315
This patient complains of severe unremitting headache, excessive sweating and pins and needles in his hands and forearms.

a What diagnosis is suggested by the radiological appearance of his hands?
b What is the likely cause of his paraesthesiae?

314
315

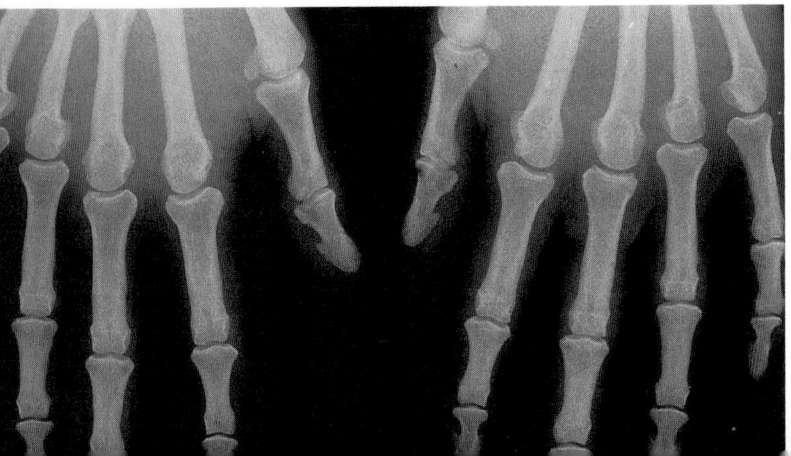

316

This twenty year old patient has a refractory error.

a What name is given to the abnormal fundal appearance?

b Is the eyeball likely to be abnormally long or abnormally short?

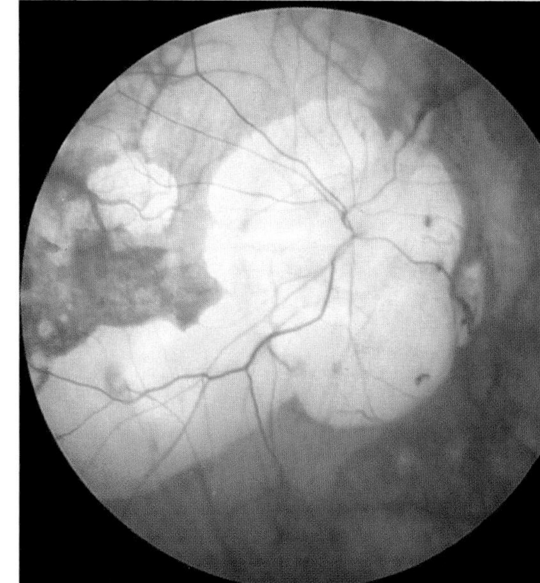

316
317

317

This patient has recently been aware of flu-like symptoms. Two weeks ago she developed a generalised rash. She has generalised lymphadenopathy and her blood pressure is 190/120. Urine microscopy reveals red cells and red cell casts.

a What is the underlying diagnosis?

b What abnormality would you expect on renal biopsy?

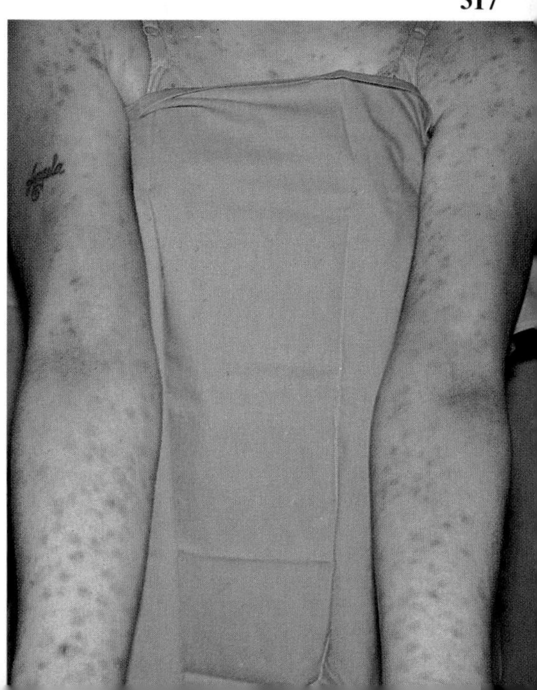

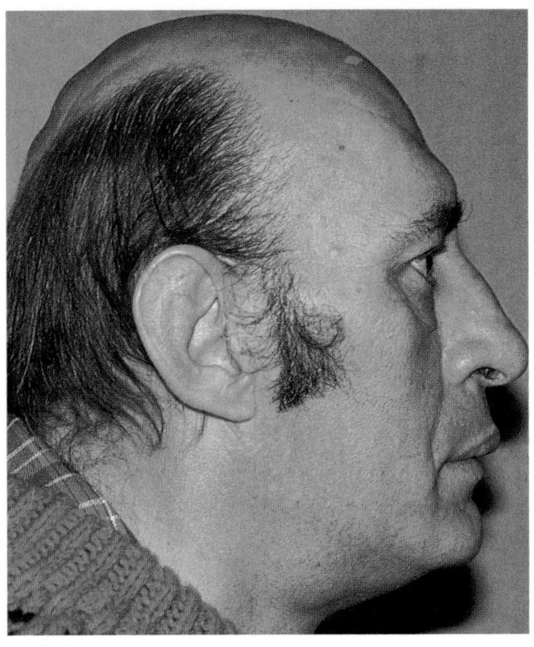

318

318
This man is acromegalic. Name five abnormalities which may be seen on a lateral skull x-ray.

319
This elderly patient lives alone, and has 'gone off her legs'. There is no history of fall, other injury or clinical evidence of a haemorrhagic diathesis. She has a normochromic anaemia, with normal white cell and platelet counts. The Hess test is positive.

a What is the likely cause of the bruising seen here?
b She is edentulous. Would you expect to find evidence of the above condition in her gums?
c How is the diagnosis established biochemically?

319

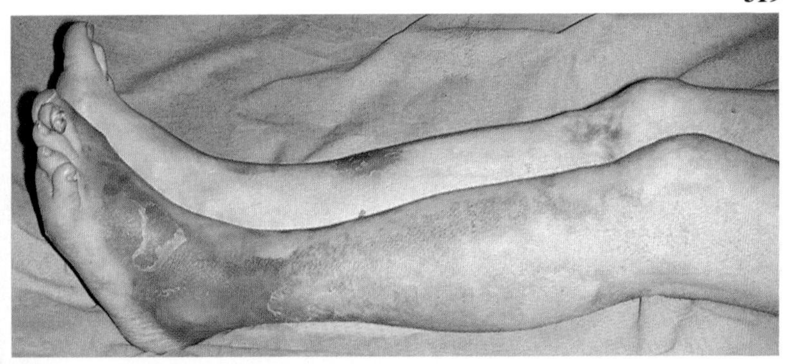

320

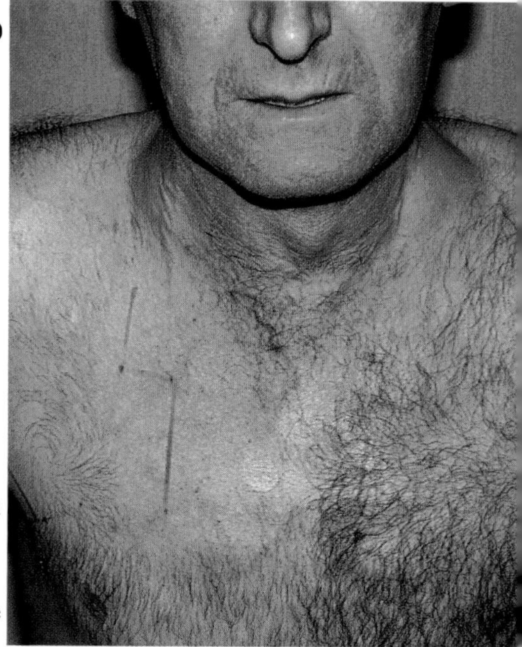

320 and 321

This patient complains of headache on awakening in the morning, of one week's duration.

a What abnormalities are seen on
  i) his chest wall?
  ii) his chest x-ray?

b What is the cause of his symptoms and what is the most likely diagnosis?

c What treatment has he received?

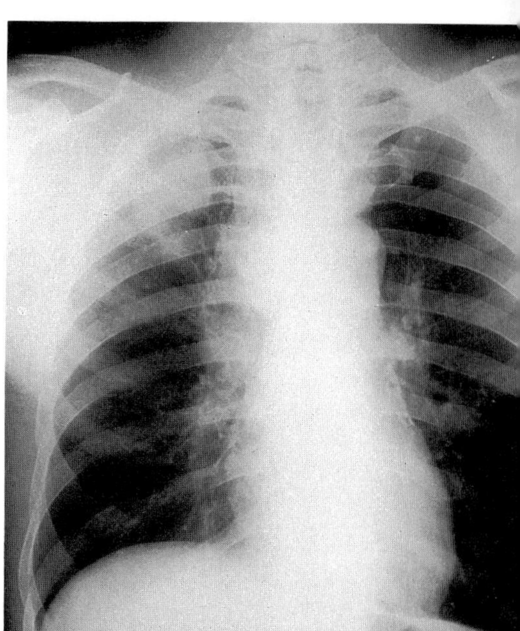

321

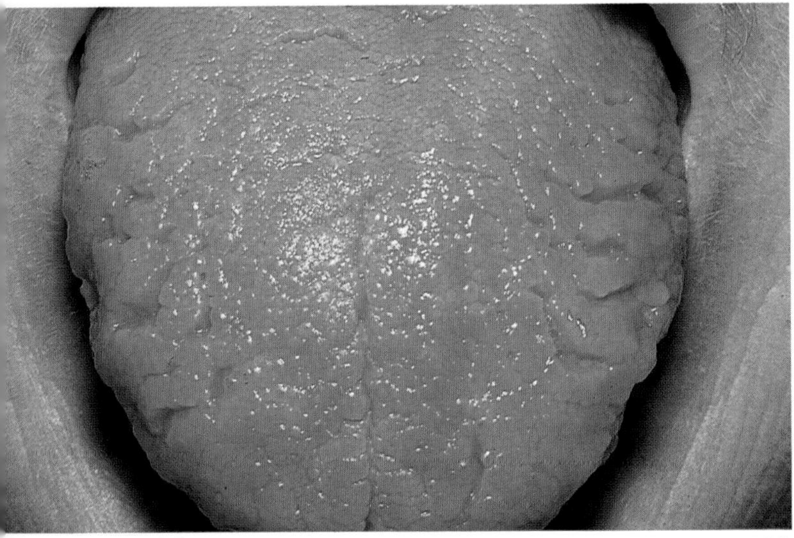

322

322 This woman experiences recurrent swelling of her lips.
a What abnormality is shown?
b What else is she likely to suffer from?
c What is this condition called?

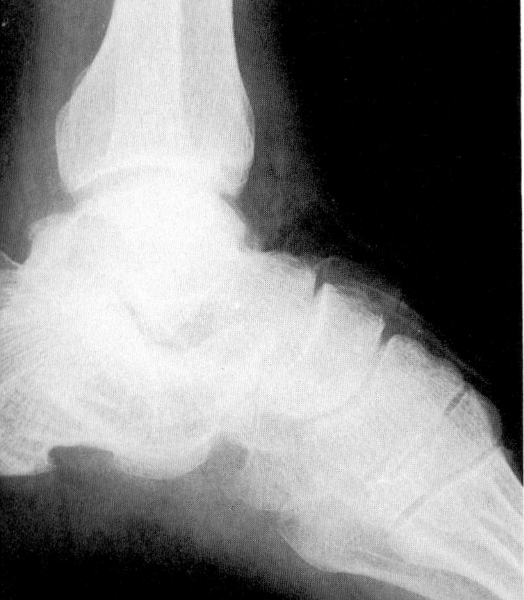

323

323
This diabetic patient has severe peripheral vascular disease. Following minor trauma to a toenail, he has experienced increasingly severe pain in the forefoot.
a What radiological abnormality is visible?
b What is the diagnosis?

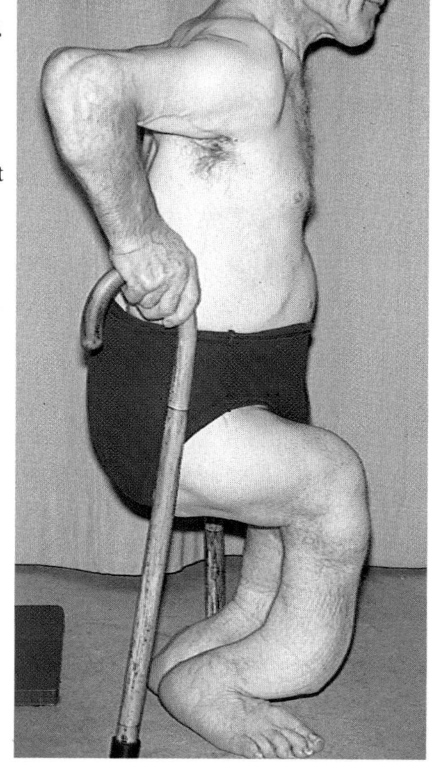

324

324 This patient's sclerae are white. Recently he has complained of increased swelling of the lower right tibia, with intense pain locally.

a What is the underlying diagnosis?

b What complication has developed?

325 This woman has normal vision.

a What is this lesion?

b What treatment is indicated?

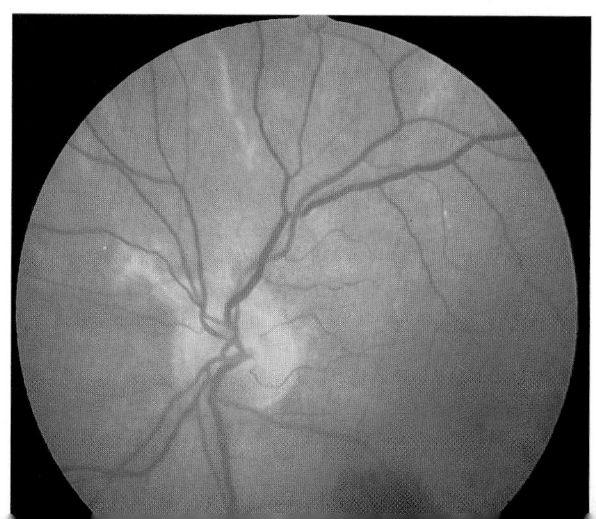

325

326

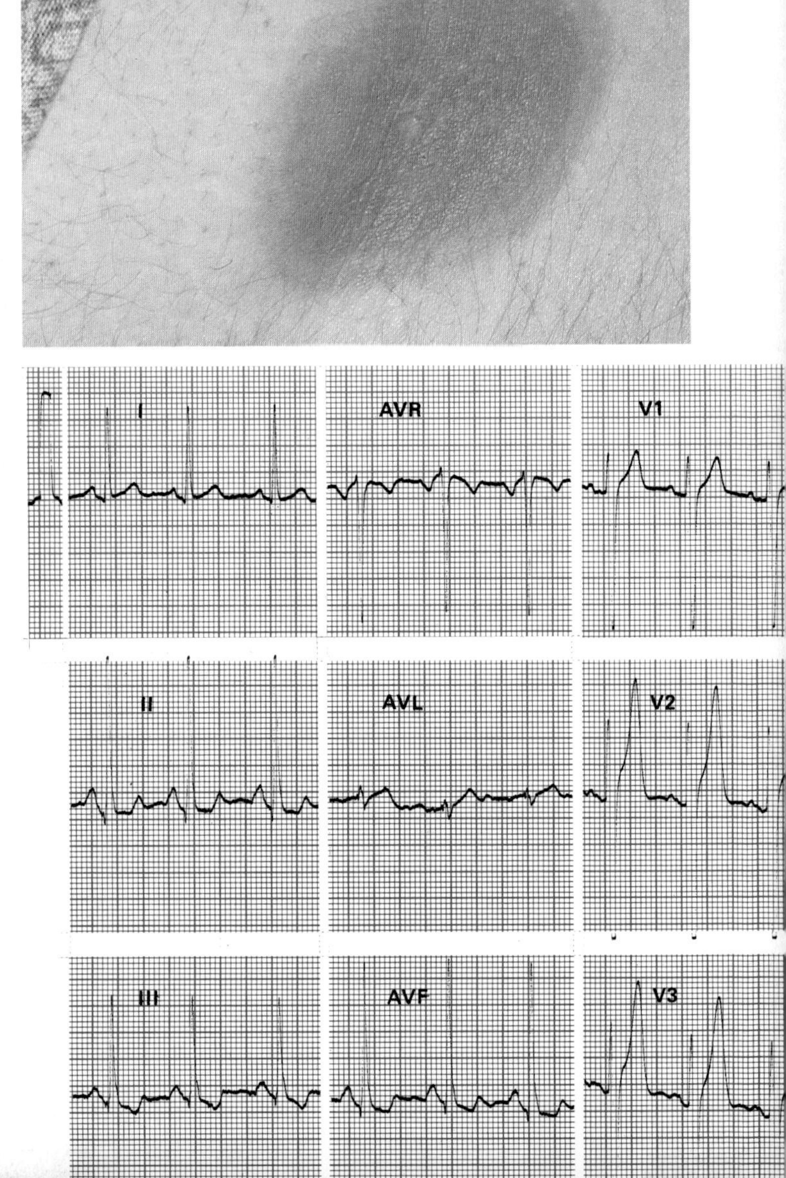

For hypertension,

These calcium channel blockers are dihydropyridines

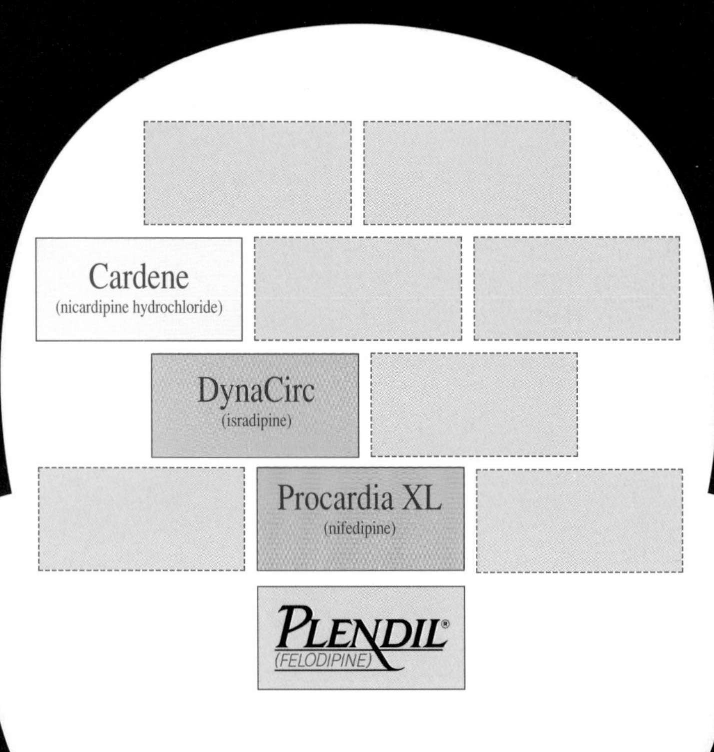

Only two dihydropyridine calcium channel blockers offer once-a-day dosing

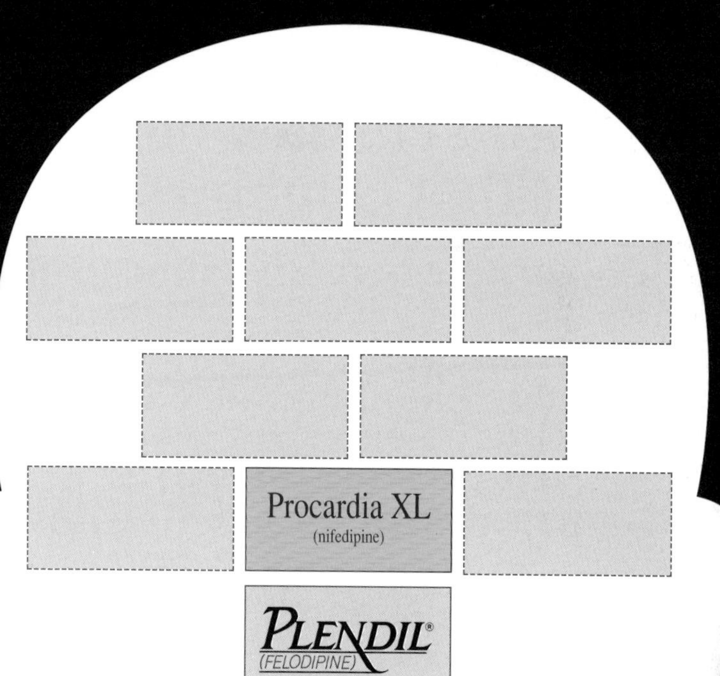

Please see the Prescribing Information on the last pages of this book.

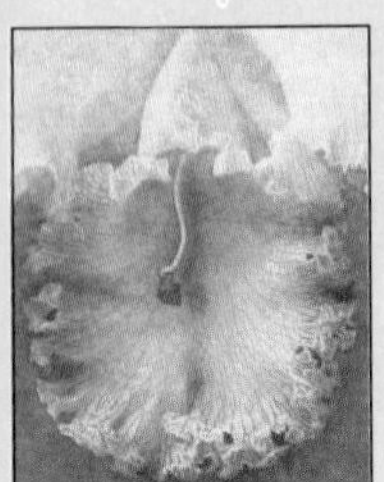

For mild-to-moderate hypertension

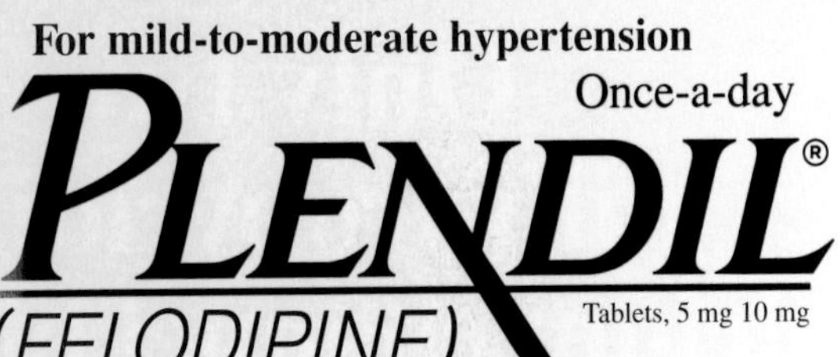

For many appropriate patients,

A vascular-selective dihydropyridine calcium channel blocker that combines

- **a favorable hemodynamic profile**
- **highly effective 24-hour blood pressure control**
- **savings from 26% to 59% compared with the starting doses of other once-a-day calcium channel blockers***

PLENDIL is contraindicated in patients who are hypersensitive to this product. Felodipine, like other calcium antagonists, may occasionally precipitate significant hypotension and, rarely, syncope. It may lead to reflex tachycardia, which in susceptible individuals may precipitate angina pectoris. (See ADVERSE REACTIONS.)

Although acute hemodynamic studies in a small number of patients with NYHA Class II or III heart failure treated with felodipine have not demonstrated negative inotropic effects, safety in patients with heart failure has not been established. Caution, therefore, should be exercised when using PLENDIL in patients with heart failure or compromised ventricular function, particularly in combination with a beta blocker.

*Based on the usual recommended starting dose(s) from the manufacturers' current product information for once-a-day calcium channel blockers for hypertension. Prices are manufacturers' direct prices, if available, or average wholesale prices from *MEDI-SPAN® Prescription Pricing Guide*, November 1992, based on the package size with the lowest per tablet cost for each strength.

Tomorrow's Horizon
A/M GROUP of MERCK & CO. Inc

Please see the Prescribing Information on the last pages of this book.

326
This lesion developed during an exacerbation of chronic obstructive airways disease. It has also appeared during earlier exacerbations, but has always healed, leaving only minimal pigmentation.

a What is the diagnosis?
b What are the two most likely causes in this patient?
c How would you establish the diagnosis?

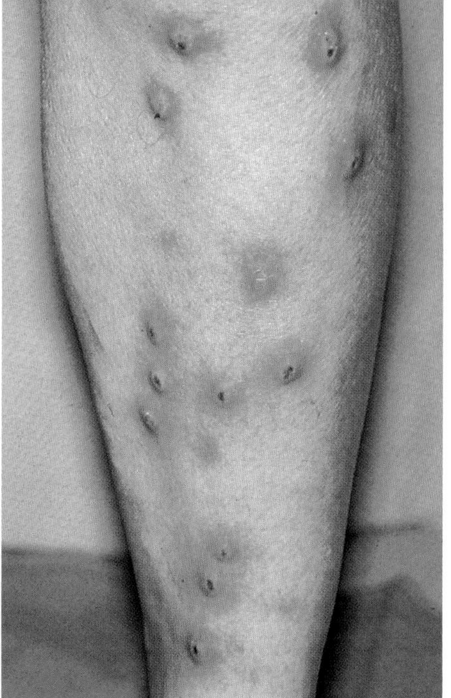

328

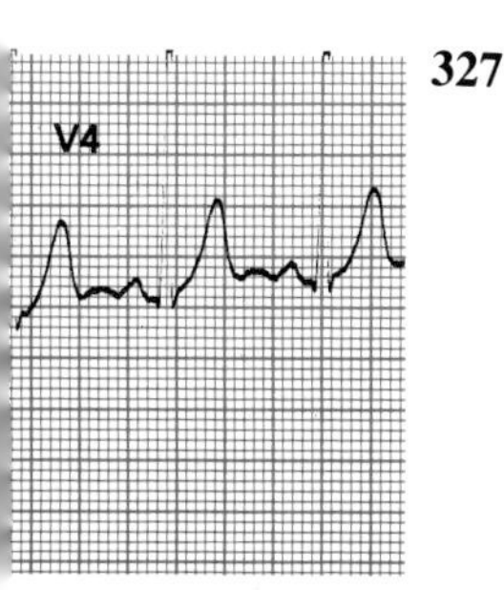

327

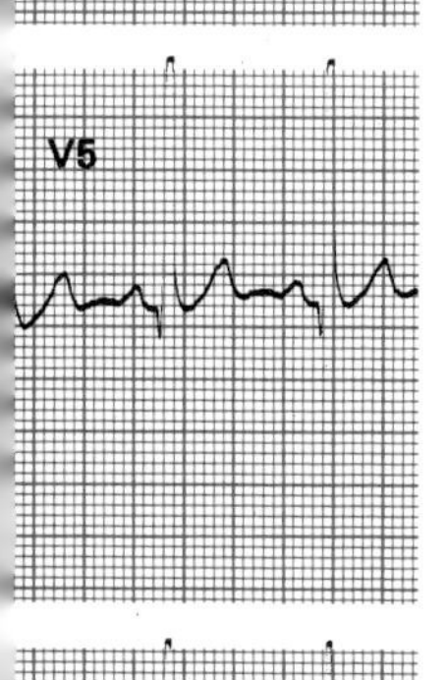

328 This forty-five year old woman complains of intense pruritus of both shins. She dates the symptoms from a visit to her local cinema two years ago.

a What is the diagnosis?
b What form of therapy is usually successful?

327 This is the ECG of a thirty year old man admitted for investigation of dyspepsia.
What immediate action should be taken?

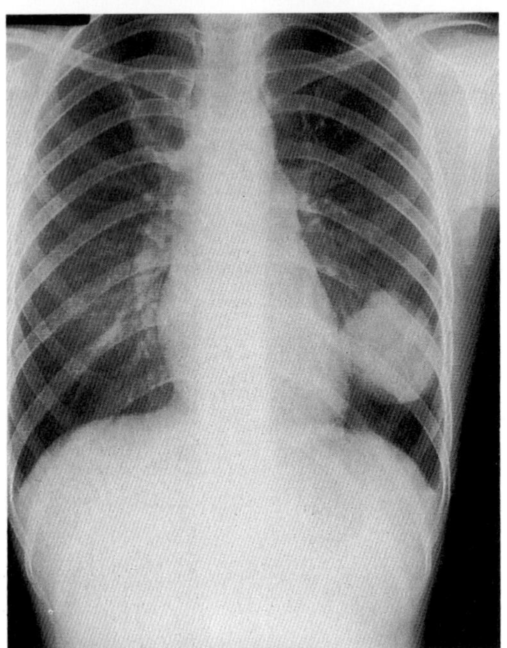

329
This shepherd suffers from a disease which has been eradicated from Iceland.

a What is the diagnosis?
b What is the distribution of this disease throughout the world?
c What is man's rôle in the life-cycle of this disease?

329

330 a What is this condition?
b Which three groups of drugs are commonly responsible for its development?

330

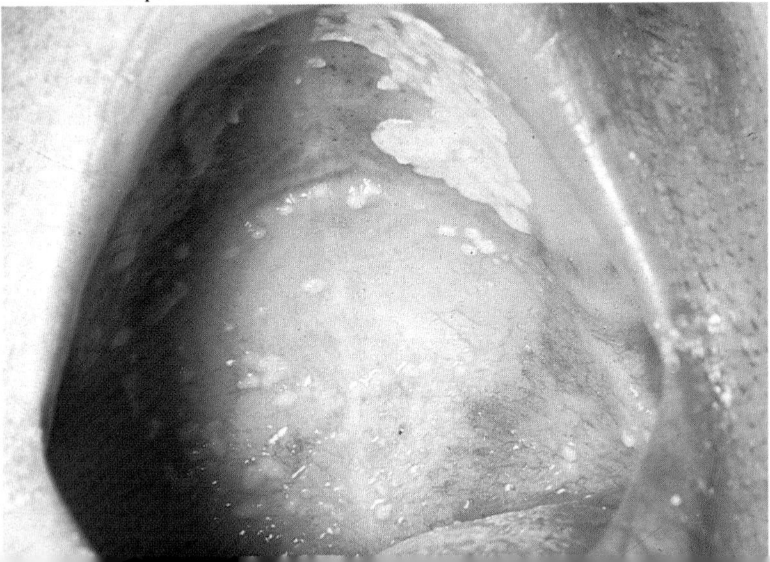

331

a What investigation is this?

b What abnormality is present?

c What neurological abnormalities are typical of this condition?

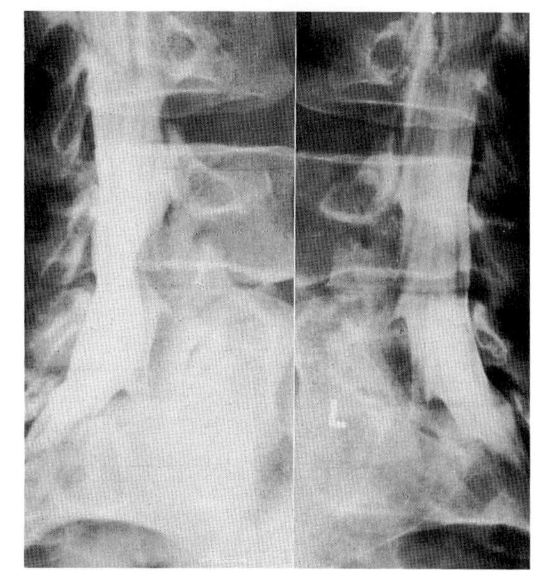

331

332

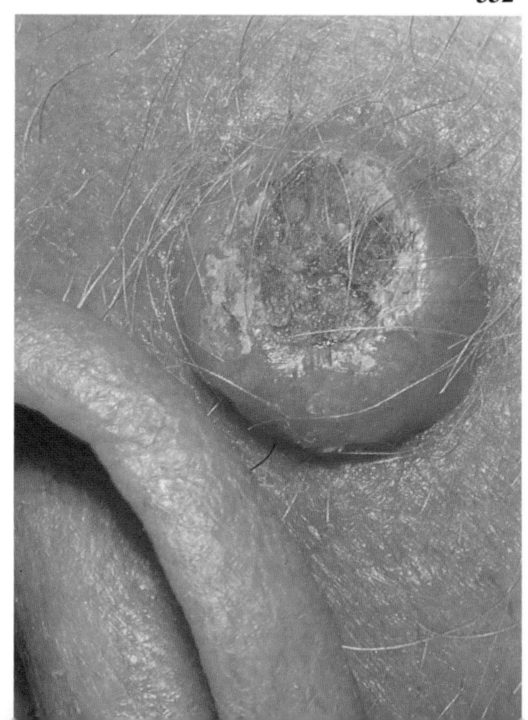

332

a What is the most likely cause of the lesion seen behind this patient's ear?

b Would you expect to find submandibular lymphadenopathy?

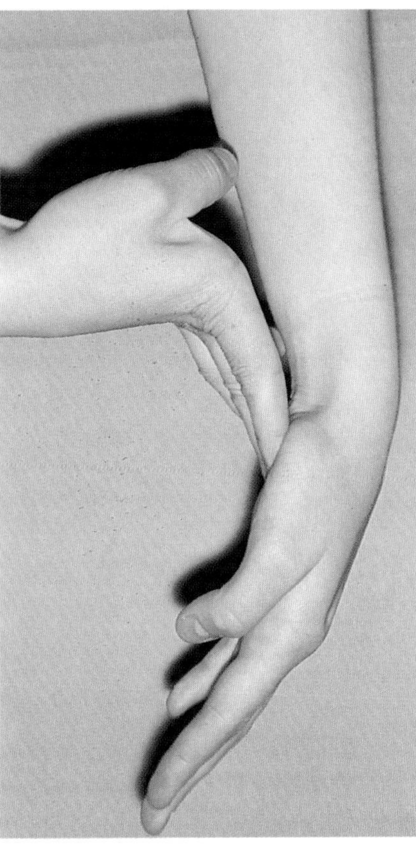

333

333 and 334 This patient has been found to have an apical midsystolic murmur on routine clinical examination.

a What abnormalities are seen of
   i) the forearms?
   ii) the skin?

b What is the diagnosis?

c Which cardiac valvular abnormality, associated with this condition, explains the murmur?

334

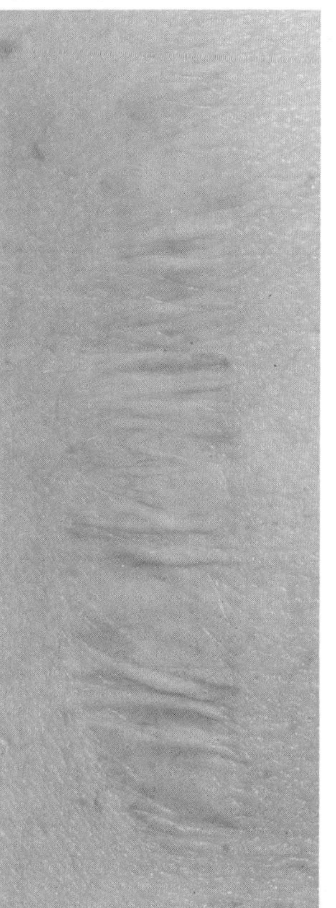

335

This woman is free of symptoms and is on no regular medication.

a What is the most likely cause of her skin pigmentation?

b In what other sites would you expect to find pigmentation in this condition?

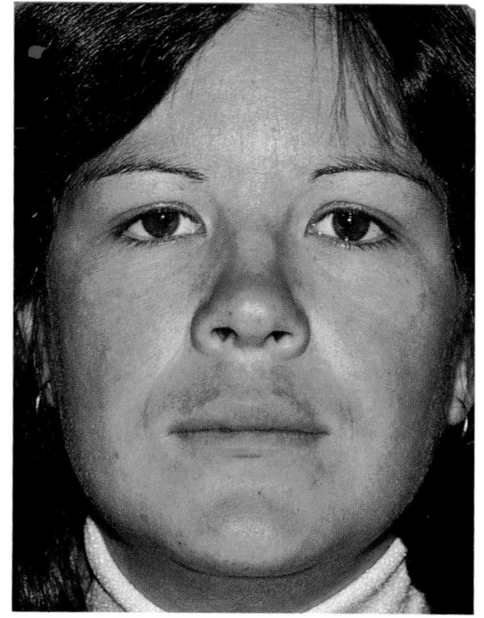

335

336

This patient had an appendicectomy two years ago. She now complains of general malaise of indeterminate onset.

a What abnormality of the appendicectomy scar can be seen?

b What diagnosis does this suggest?

c What information does the scar give about onset of this disorder?

336

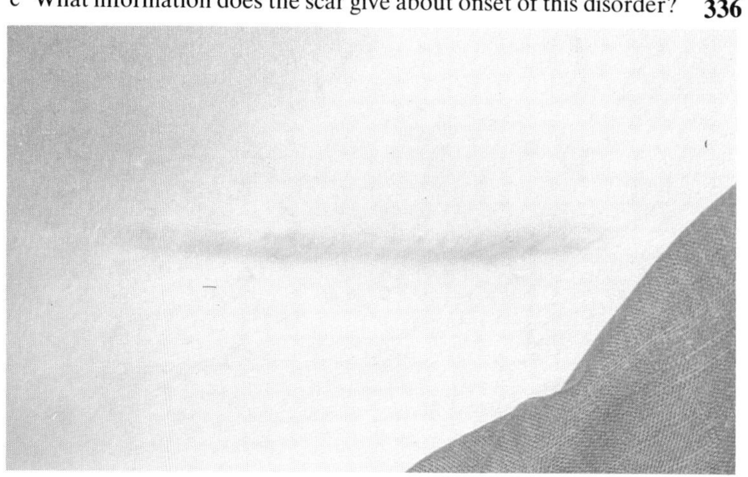

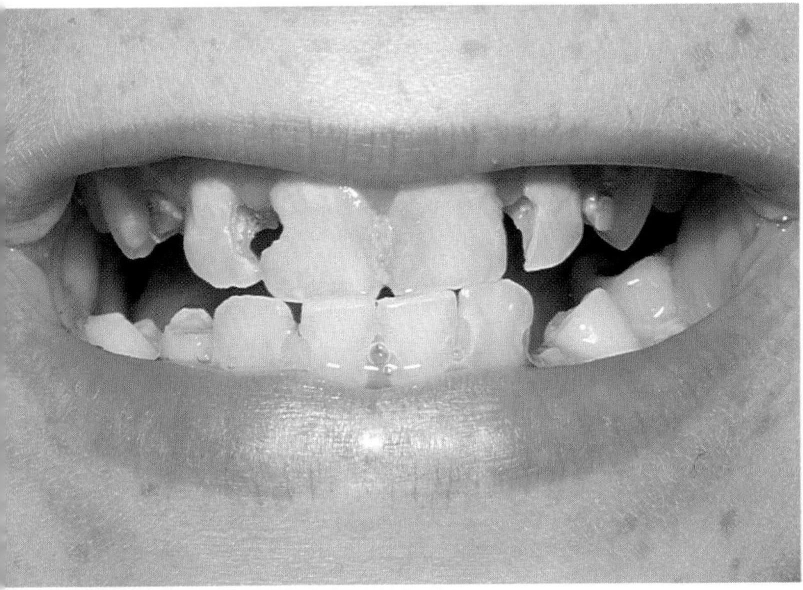

337

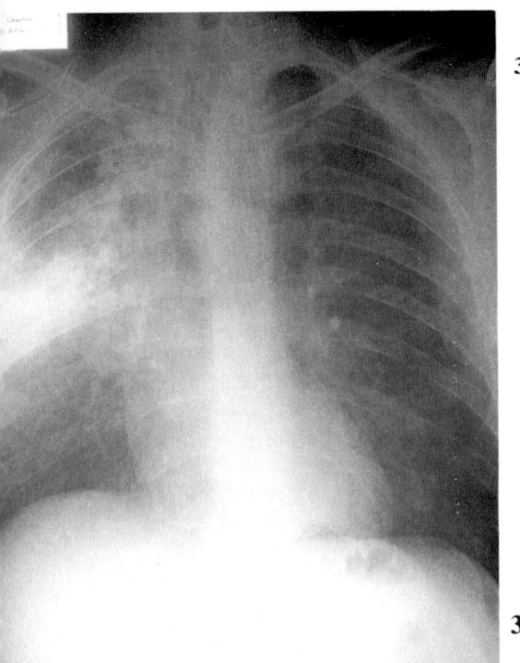

337 and 338 This young man presented with chronic cough, purulent sputum and weight loss. Examination of sputum revealed the presence of sulphur granules.

a What is the diagnosis?
b Which serological test is useful in confirming the diagnosis?
c What is the significance of his dental hygiene?

338

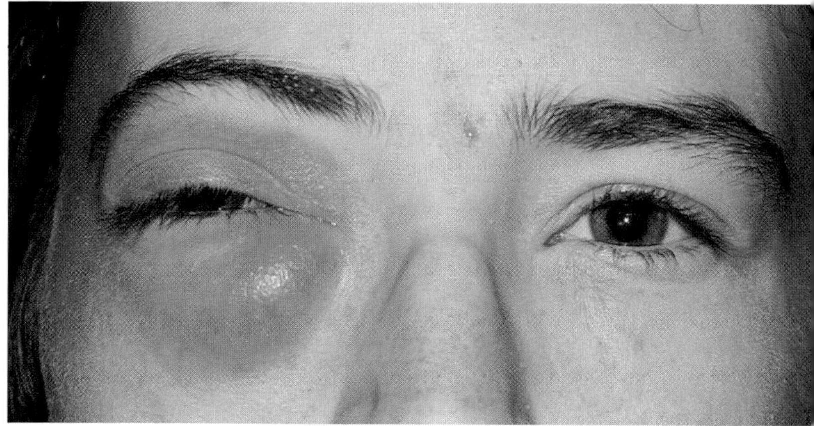

339 a What is this condition?
b What complications may develop?
c What signs would indicate involvement of the globe?

339

340
This woman complained of severe pain in her left forearm and hand for three days. She then developed this vesicular, crusted eruption.
a What is the diagnosis?
b Which nerve roots are affected?

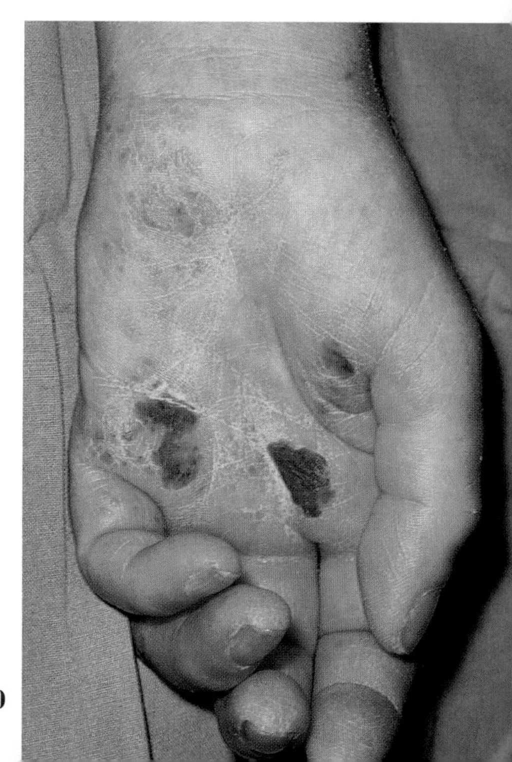

340

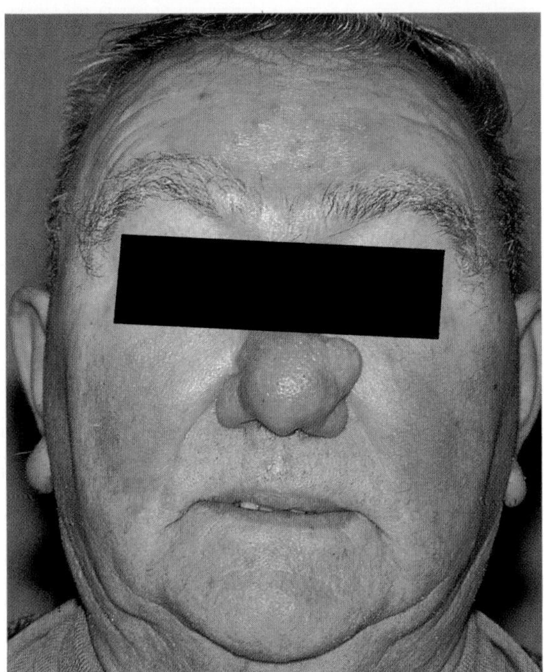

341

341

a What is the most likel
cause of this patient's facial rash?

b List four ocular complications of this disorder.

342

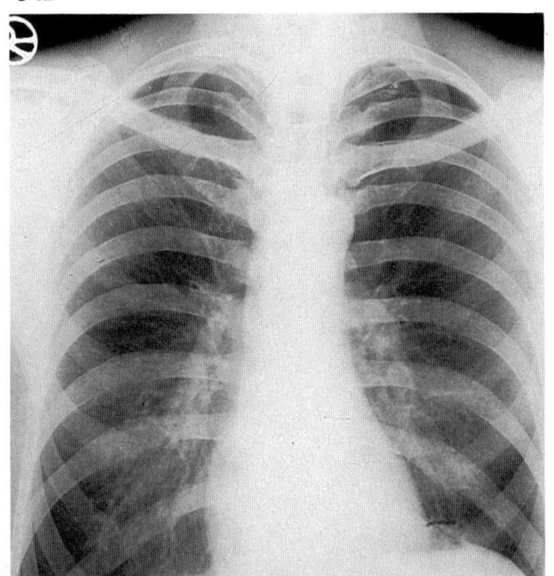

342

This young patient presents with sudden onset of pleuritic chest pain and breathlessness

What abnormality is seen on chest x-ray?

343

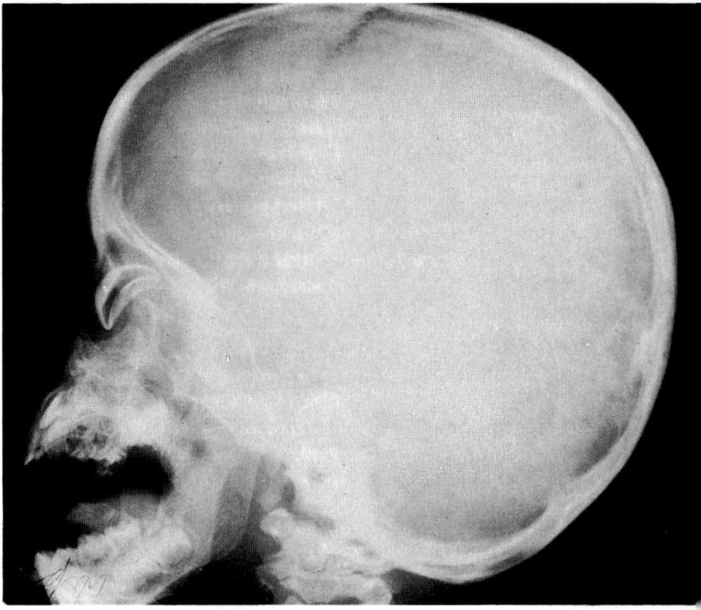

343

This patient is jaundiced.

a What abnormality is seen in the lateral skull x-ray?

b How does this explain his jaundice?

344

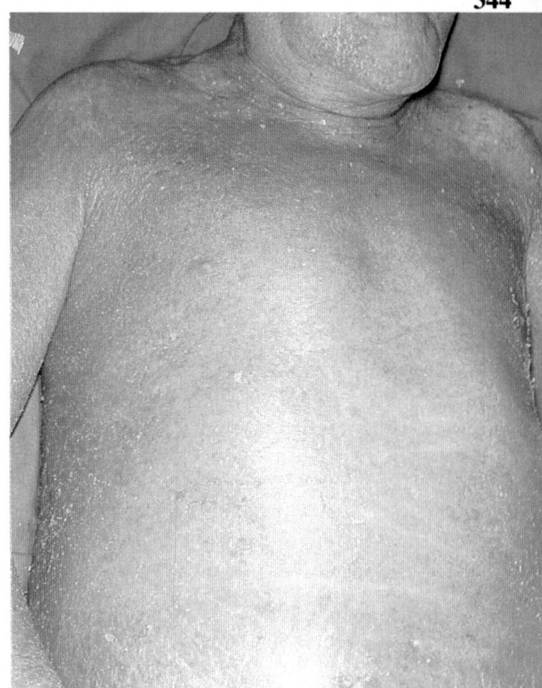

344

This patient complains of generalised intense pruritus. In addition to the skin abnormality, he has generalised lymphadenopathy. He is taking no drugs and there is no history of previous skin disorder.

a What dermatological abnormality is seen?

b What underlying systemic diseases should be considered?

c List four complications of the skin disorder.

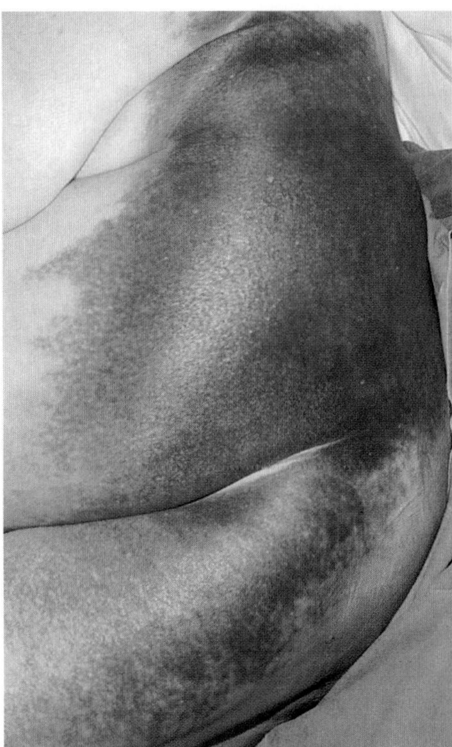

345

346

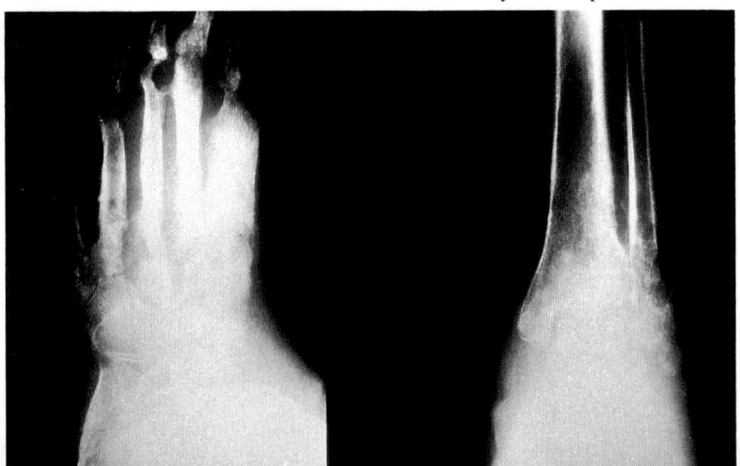

345
This woman has a family history of bleeding and a lifelong personal history of recurrent epistaxis and menorrhagia.
a What is the likely diagnosis?
b What will the bleeding time show?
c What will the result be of platelet aggregation studies with collagen?
d What percentage of her children will be affected?

346
This Indian patient presented with painless swelling of his foot, with multiple draining sinuses from which black granules are occasionally discharged.
a What is the name of this condition?
b Which antibacterial agent is usually successful?
c To which organs does systemic spread occur?

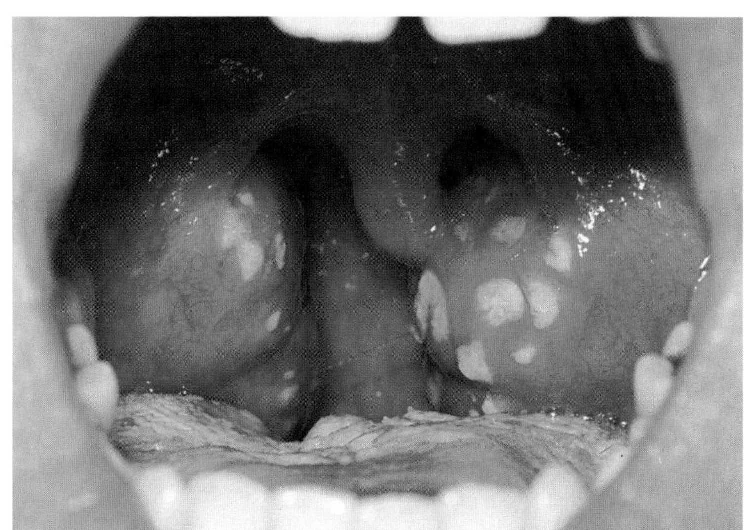

347 **347**

What signs will differentiate streptococci from viruses as a cause of this appearance?

348

348

This condition was once the healing prerogative of kings.

a What is its name?

b Which organism is usually responsible?

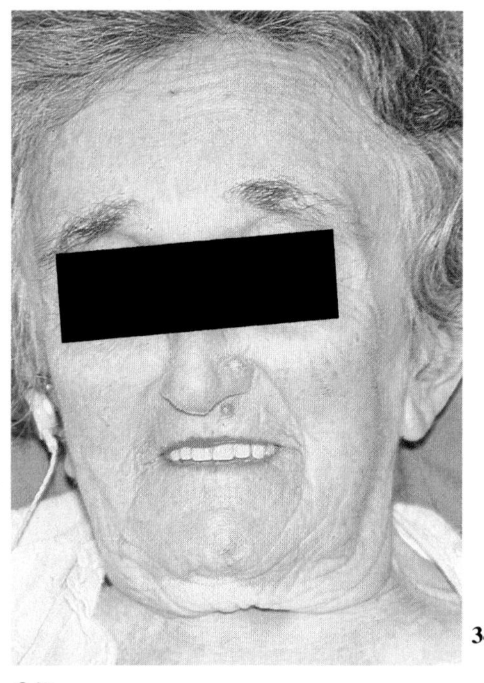

349

349 and 350

a What is the cause of this patient's deafness?

b Is specific treatment indicated?

350

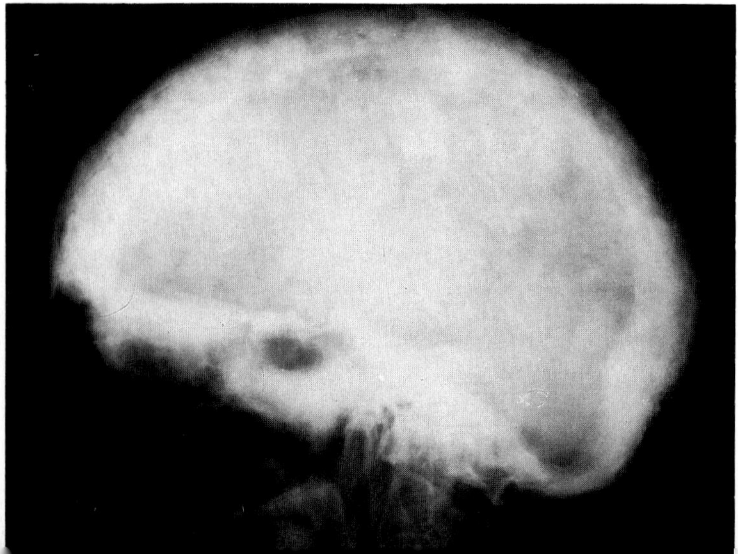

351
This patient has rheumatoid arthritis.

a What are these lesions seen near the elbow?
b What are the typical histological features of such lesions?
c With which serological abnormality are they associated?

352
This patient has raised levels of blood pressure.

a What anatomical abnormality is shown?
b What diagnosis does this suggest?
c What should be considered as a possible cause for her raised blood pressure?

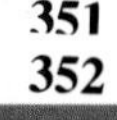

351
352

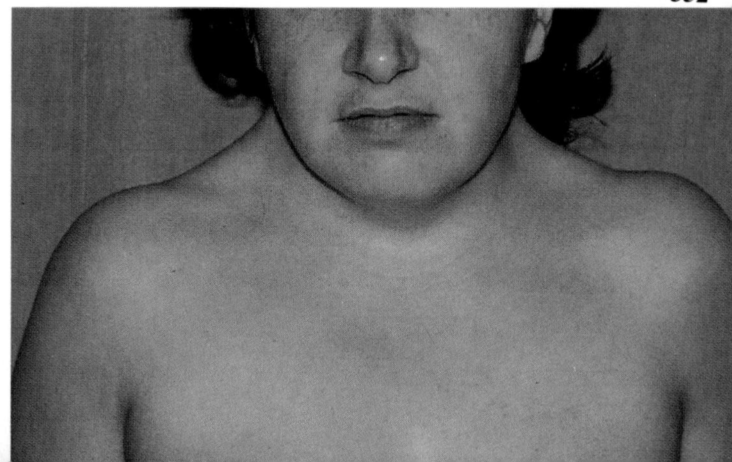

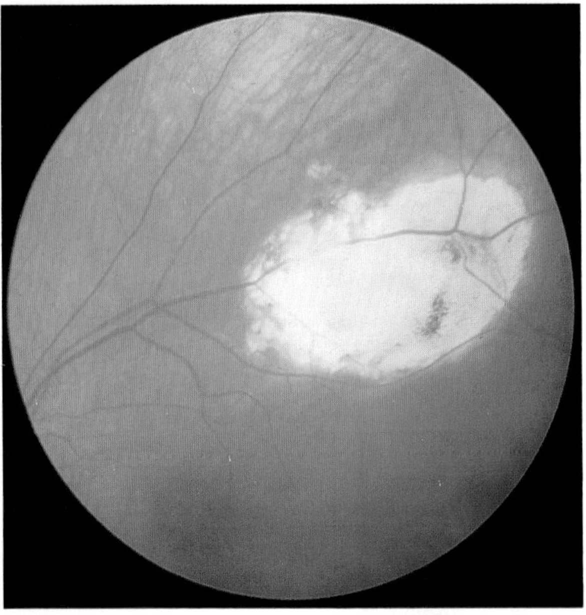

353

353 and 354

a What abnormality is shown in the
   i) fundus?
   ii) x-ray?
b How may they be associated?

354

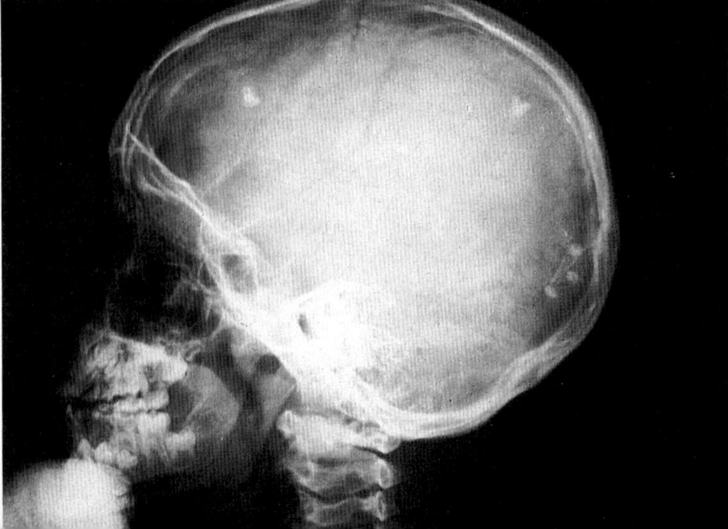

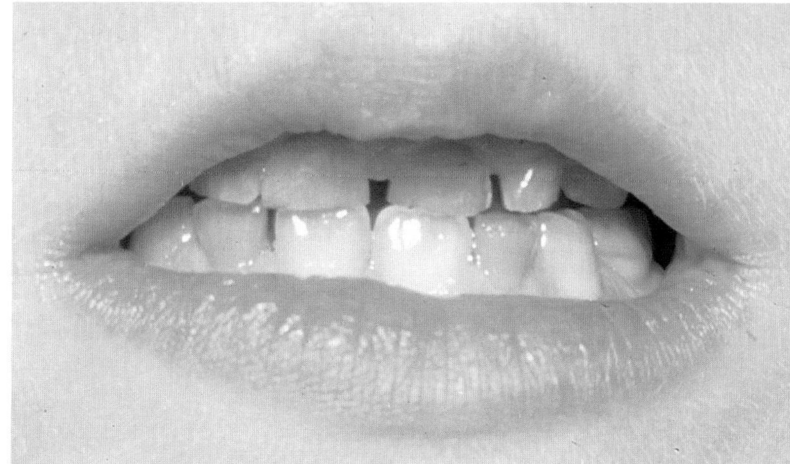

355 **355**

a What dental abnormality is present and what is the likely cause?

b How can this diagnosis be confirmed clinically?

c What is the cause of the irregularity of the appearance?

d Are these teeth more prone to caries than usual?

356

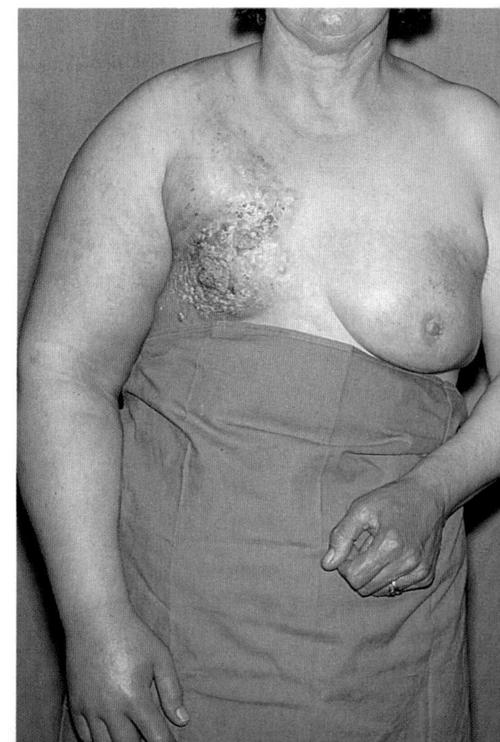

356

This woman received radiotherapy following breast surgery.

a What four abnormalities are present?

b To which rare vascular tumour may this appearance predispose?

357

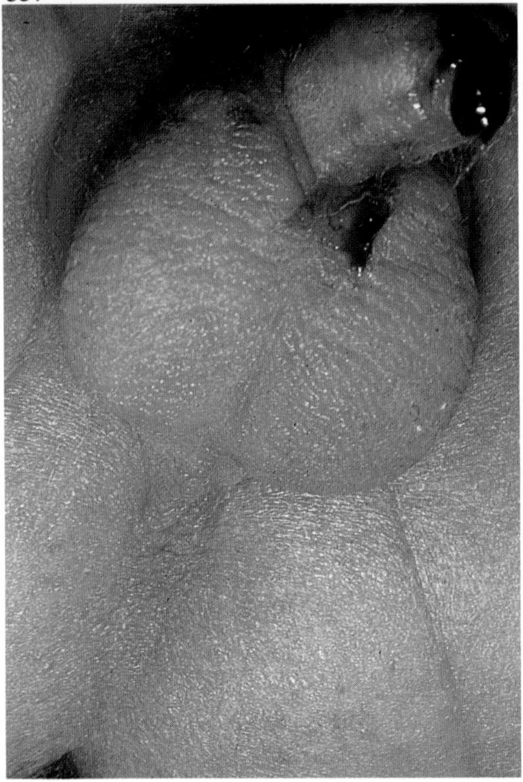

357
a What two abnormalities are present?
b What does this indicate?

359
a What is this condition?
b What underlying diagnosis should you suspect?

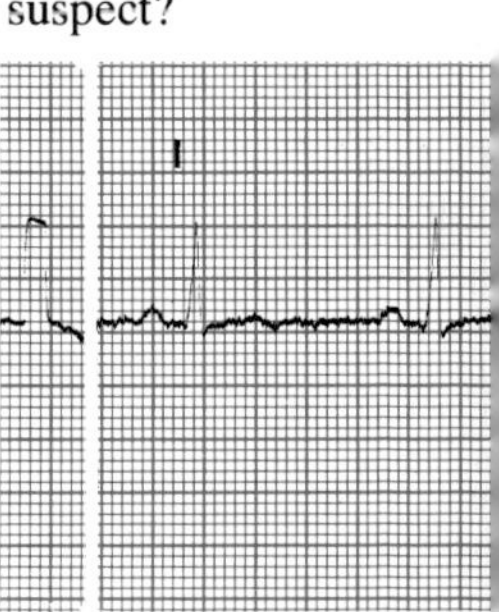

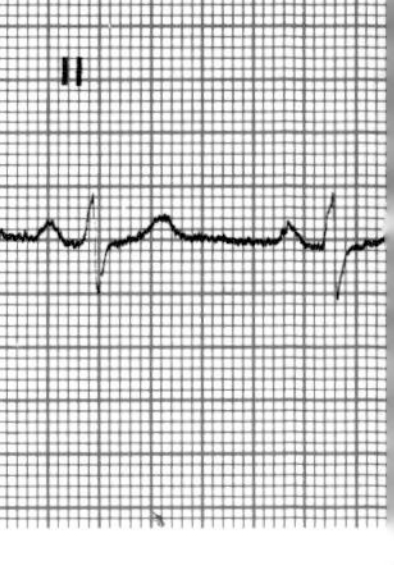

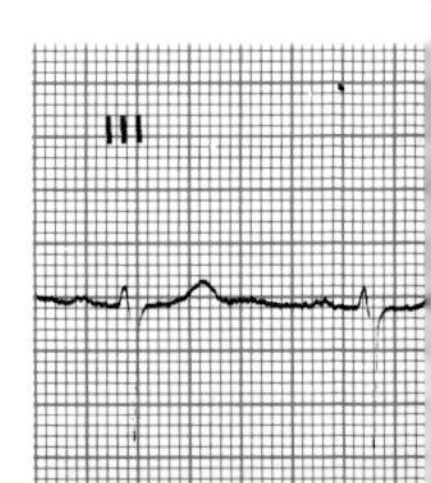

358
This middle aged man suddenly developed paralysis of his left face, arm and leg without disturbance of consciousness. Five days previously he had experienced anterior chest discomfort. Computerised tomography showed a large cerebral infarction in the territory of the right middle cerebral artery. An ECG recorded three months previously was normal.

a What is the likely cause of his stroke?
b Is immediate anticoagulation indicated?
c How might the cause of his stroke be established?

359

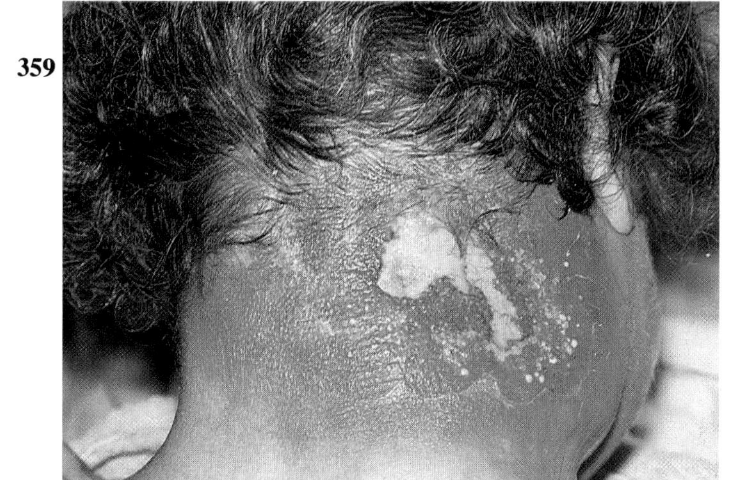

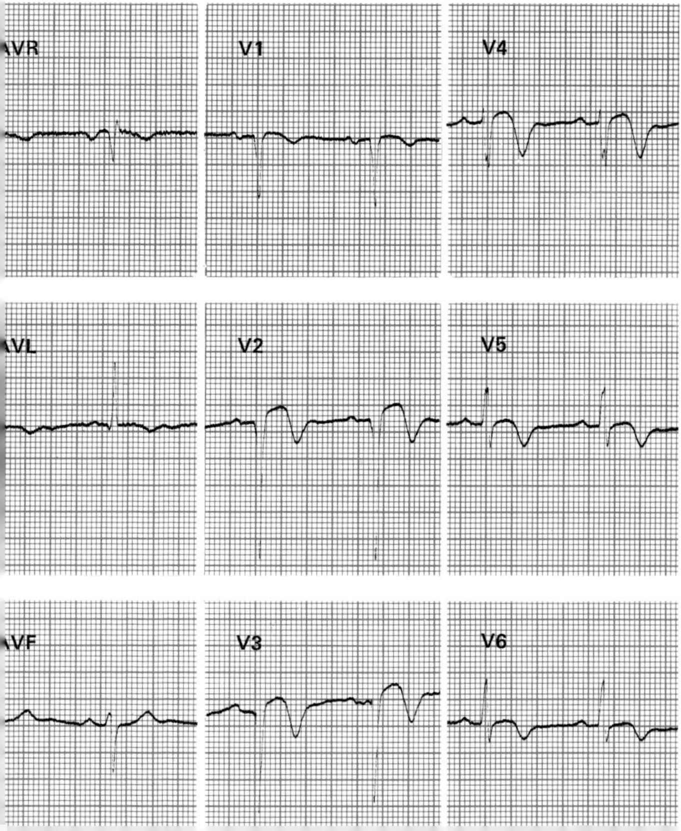

AVR V1 V4

AVL V2 V5

AVF V3 V6

358

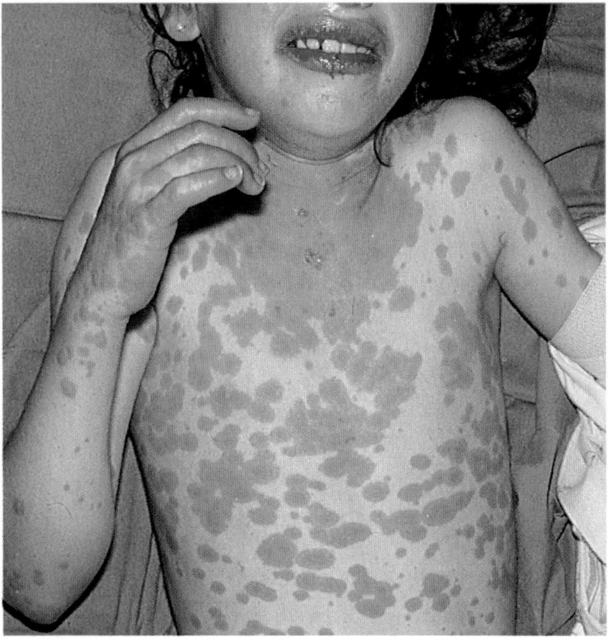

360

360 and 361

a What name is given to this girl's rash?

b Which organisms are most commonly associated with this condition?

c Are immunofluorescence studies useful in confirming the diagnosis?

361

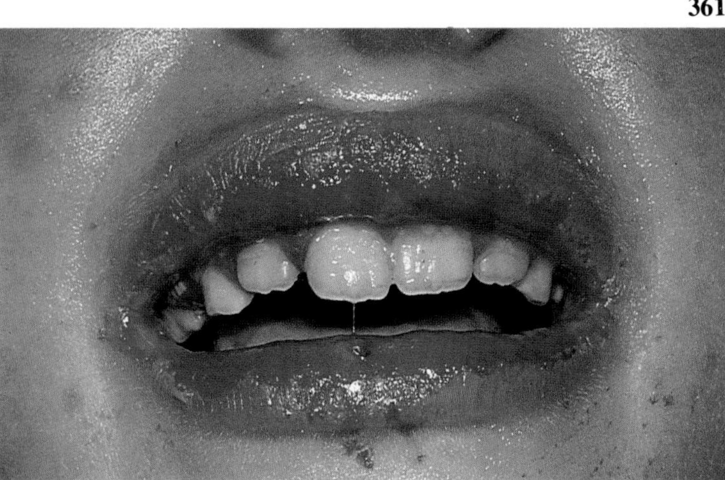

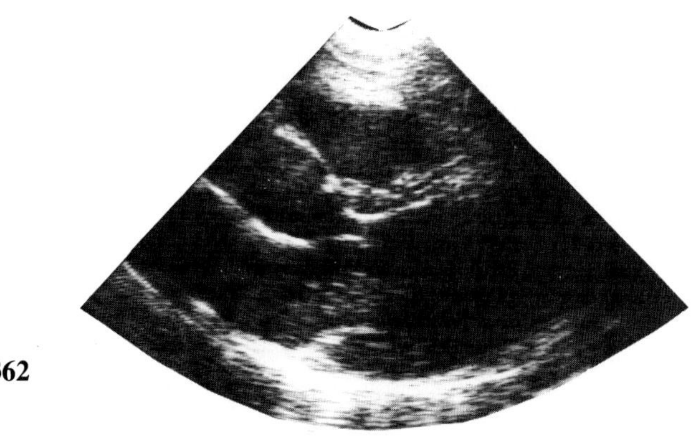

362

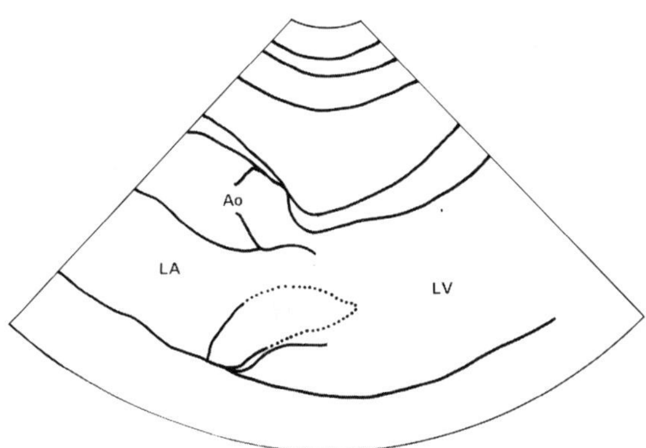

362
This forty-five year old patient presented with a two month history of malaise, weight loss and intermittent fever. There was no history of rheumatic fever in childhood. Auscultation of the heart revealed a third heart sound, with a variable relationship to the second sound and an apical pansystolic murmur. Chest x-ray showed left atrial prominence but no ventricular hypertrophy. Shortly after admission to hospital, she developed transient weakness of the right arm and leg.

a What abnormality is seen in this cross-sectional echocardiogram through the long axis of the left ventricle?
b What is the likely diagnosis?
c What treatment is necessary?

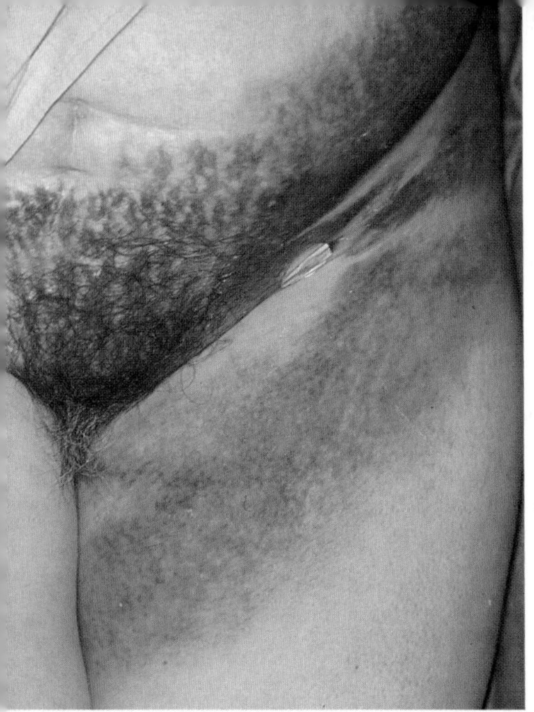

363

363

This patient, a chronic asthmatic, on regular corticosteroid treatment has been admitted to an acute medical receiving unit. The appearance shown developed shortly after admission.

What is the most likely cause of the appearance of her left groin?

364

This patient, a non-smoker, gives a six month history of night sweats and weight loss. Ten days ago she began to be aware of increasingly severe headache, worse on wakening. Her serum albumin is 35 g/l.

a What abnormality is seen?

b What is the diagnosis?

c What is the most likely underlying pathology?

d What principal abnormality would you expect to see on chest x-ray?

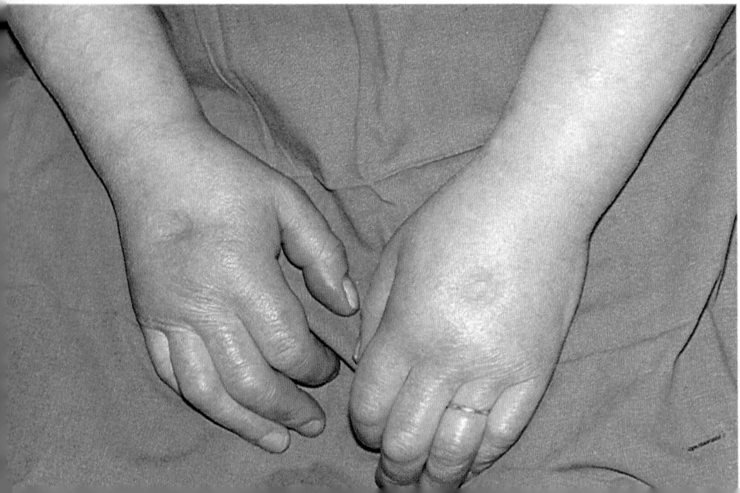

364

365
This patient complains of altered sensation in her feet, "as if walking on cotton wool".

a What two abnormalities are seen?
b What single agent may be responsible?

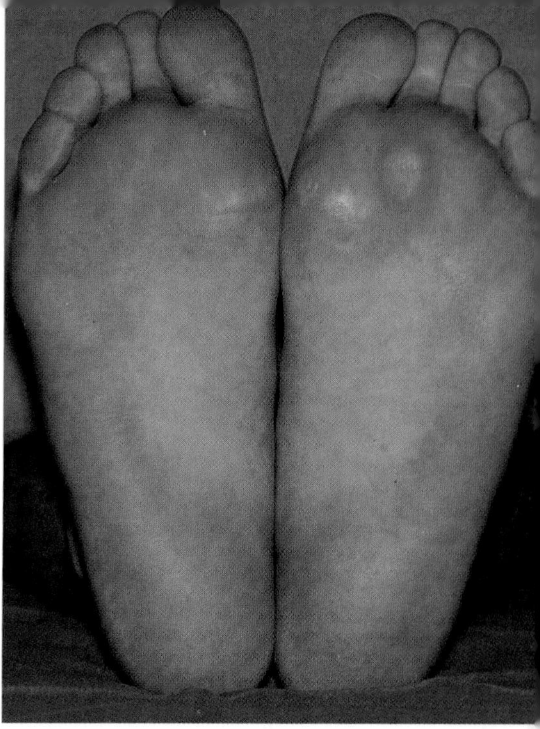

365
366

366

a What abnormalities are seen in this optic fundus?
b What investigations would you carry out to diagnose the underlying condition?

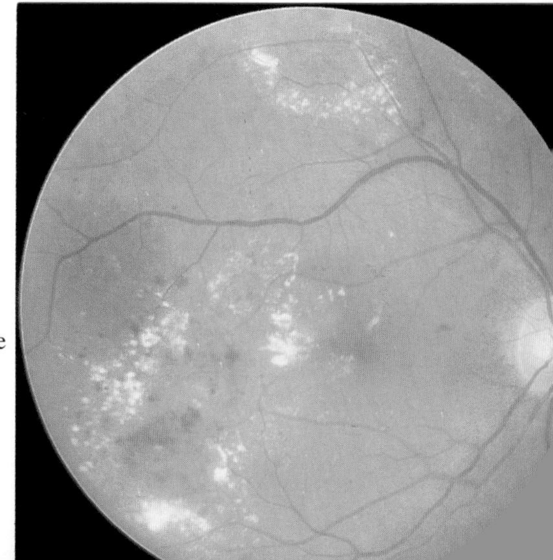

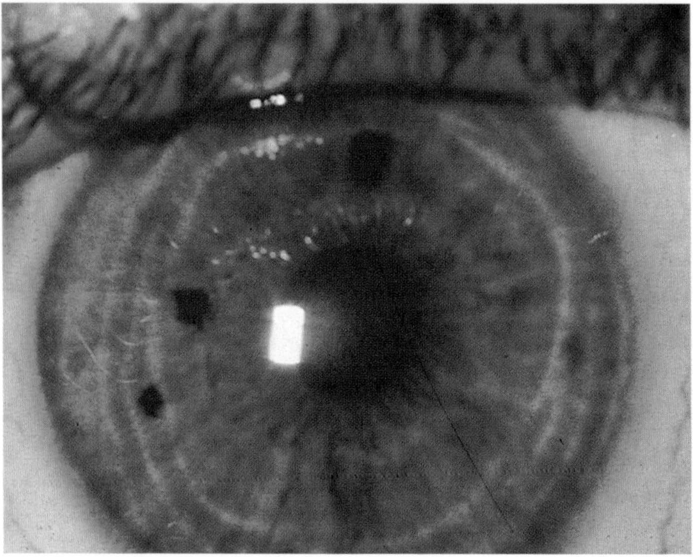

367

367 and 368 This patient has chronic renal failure. His corrected serum calcium is 3.2 mmol/l.

a What ocular abnormality is seen?

b What abnormality (apart from the acneiform rash and adhesive plaster) is seen in the picture of his chest?

c What is the likely endocrine abnormality?

368

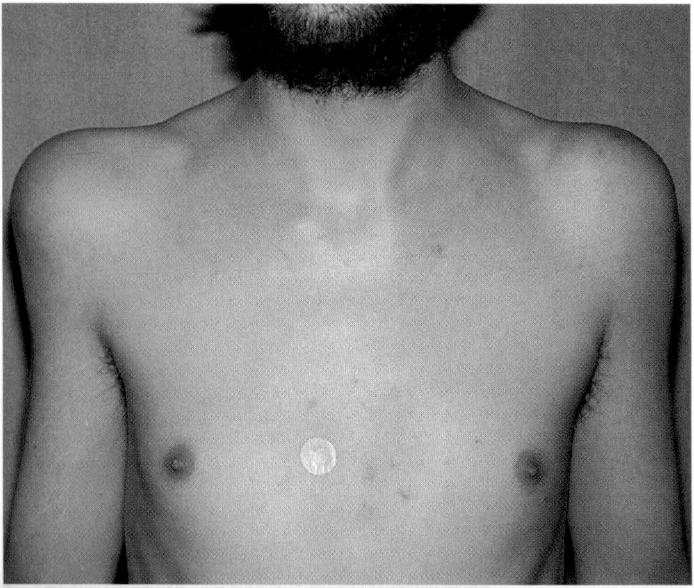

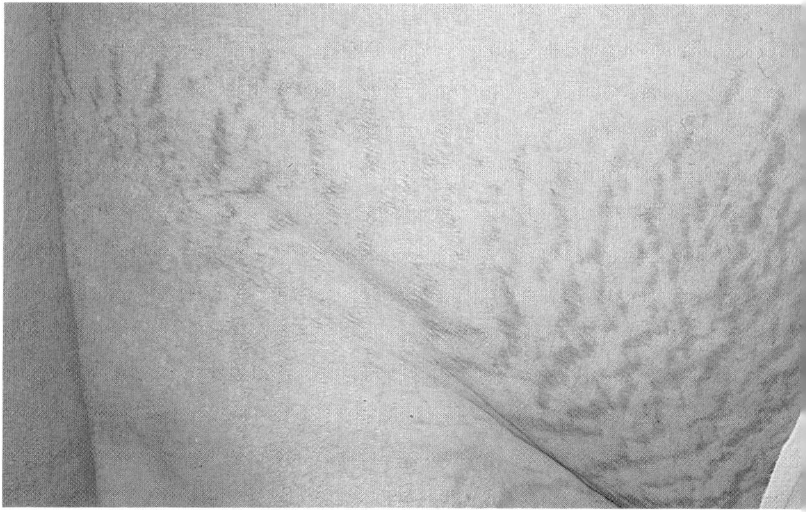

369 369

This fifty-two year old female patient is hypertensive.

a What abnormality is seen on the skin of her abdomen and thigh?

b Which underlying endocrine disorder should be considered?

c Similar skin changes may be seen in normal pregnancy. In what way do these differ in appearance from those seen in the above condition?

370

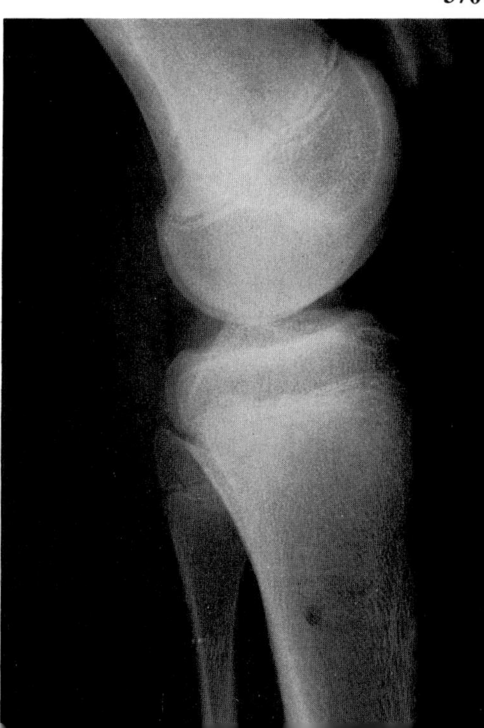

370

This eleven year old boy presented with pain and swelling around his anterior tibial tubercle.

a What radiological abnormality is present?

b What is the diagnosis?

c What treatment is required?

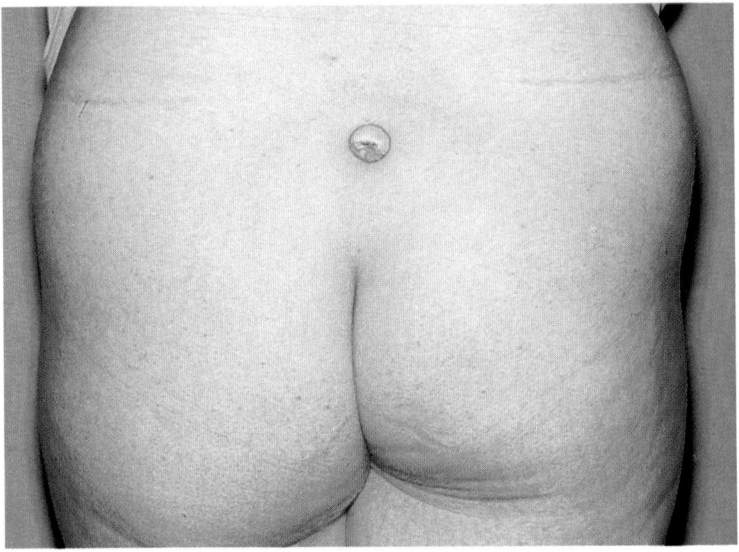

371
372

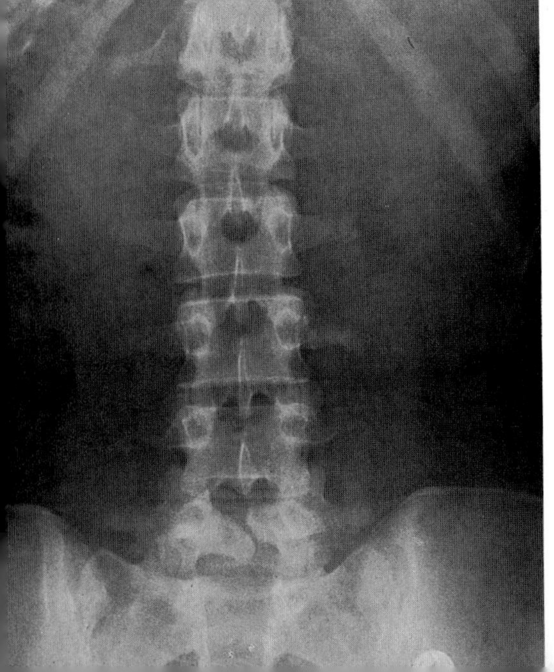

371 and 372 This teenage girl complains of occasional urinary incontinence, of recent onset. She has bilateral pes cavus and absent ankle jerks but the legs are otherwise neurologically intact.

a What is this condition?

b How does this explain her incontinence and absent ankle jerks?

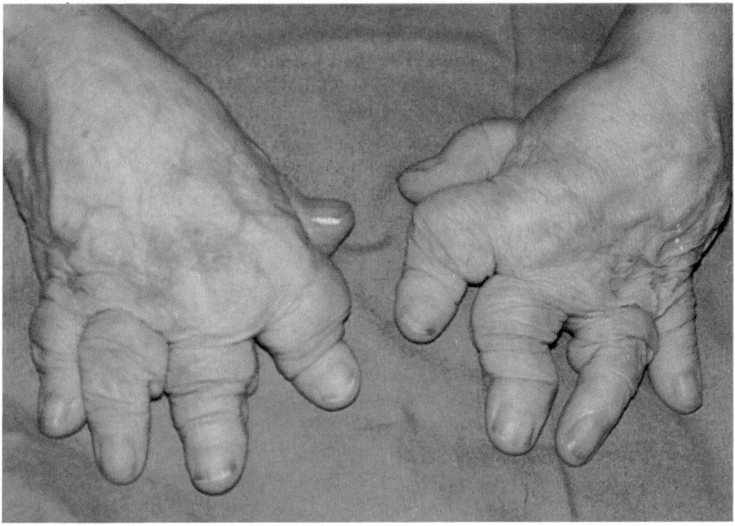

373

373 and 374 Both these patients have severe longstanding joint disease.

a What descriptive name is given to the degree of joint abnormality seen in the hands?

b Of which condition are these appearances characteristic?

c What are the three earliest radiological abnormalities in this condition?

374

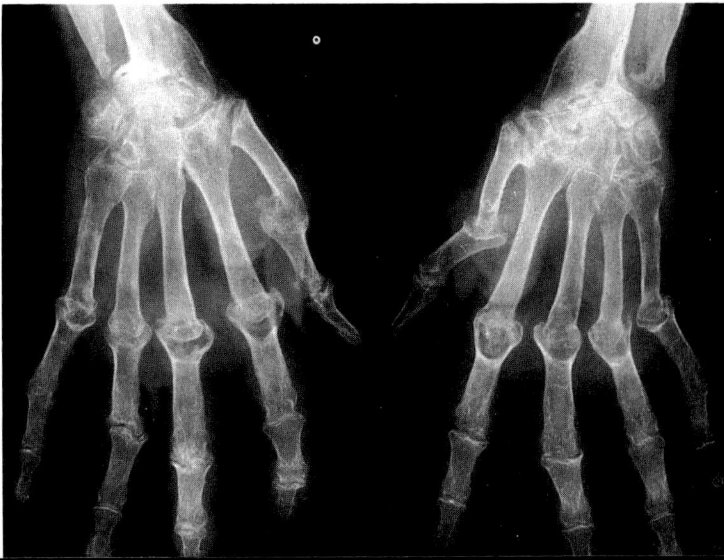

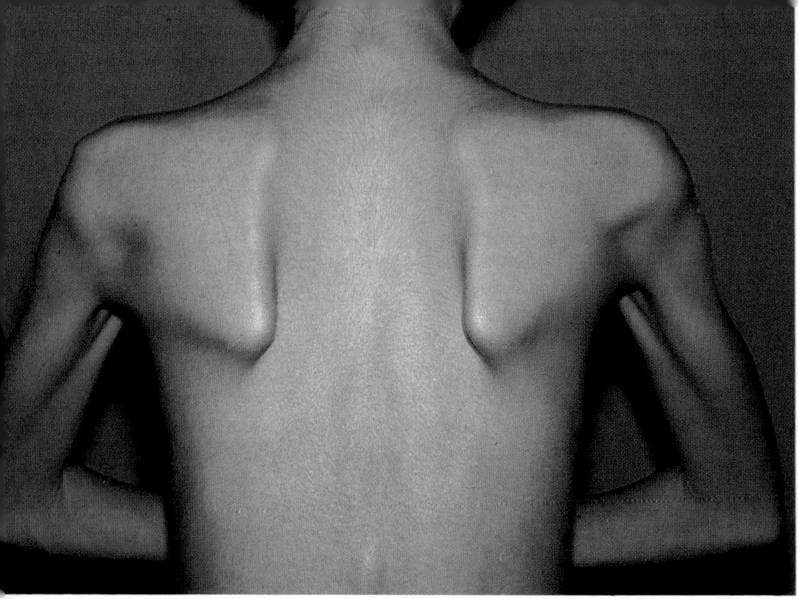

375

375, 376, 377 and 378 These patients suffer from the same progressive disorder. The first patient (whose face and back are seen) is unable to do 'press-ups' at school and cannot whistle, nor use a drinking straw. He has been asked to bare his teeth. The second patient has, in addition to severe weakness of the shoulder girdle, a high stepping gait. The third patient finds that his golf handicap is gradually increasing, but has no other complaints.

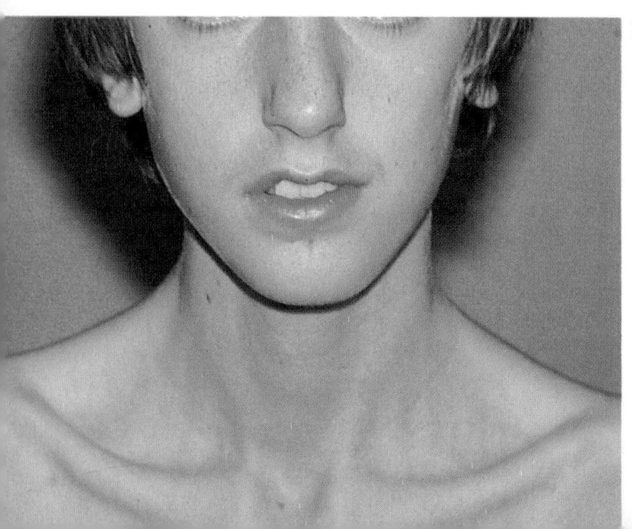

376

377

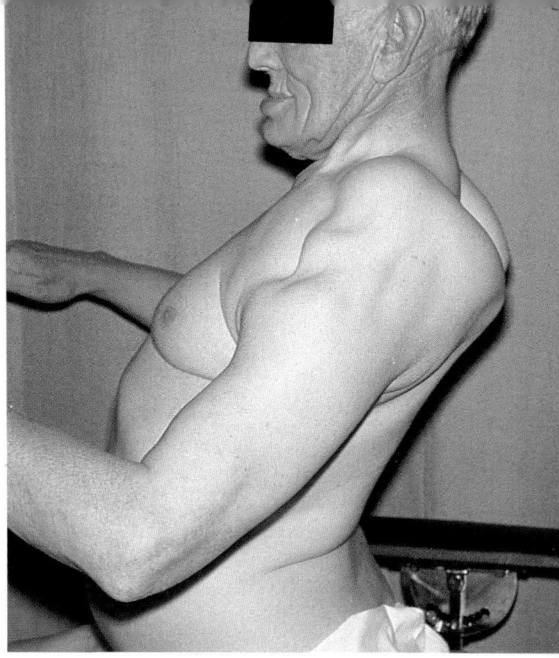

a What is the most likely diagnosis?

b i) What is the likely cause of the second patient's abnormal gait?

ii) What would you expect to find on testing his tendon reflexes?

c Which muscles are most obviously affected in

i) the first patient?

ii) the third patient?

d What effect does this disorder have on life expectancy?

378

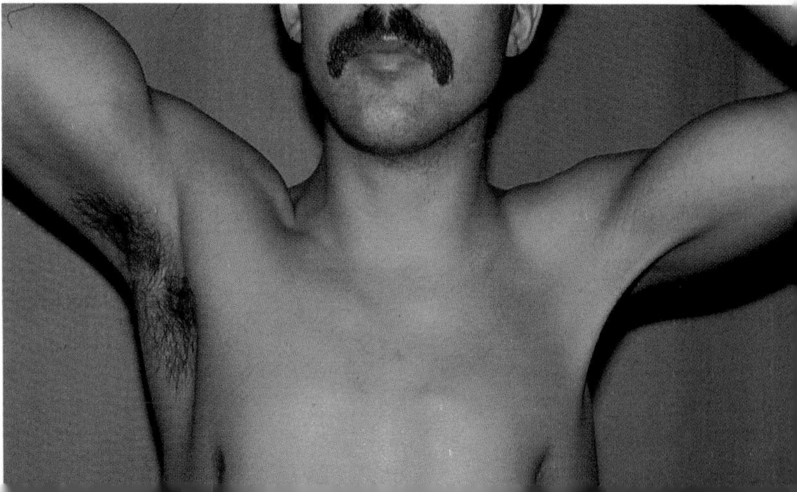

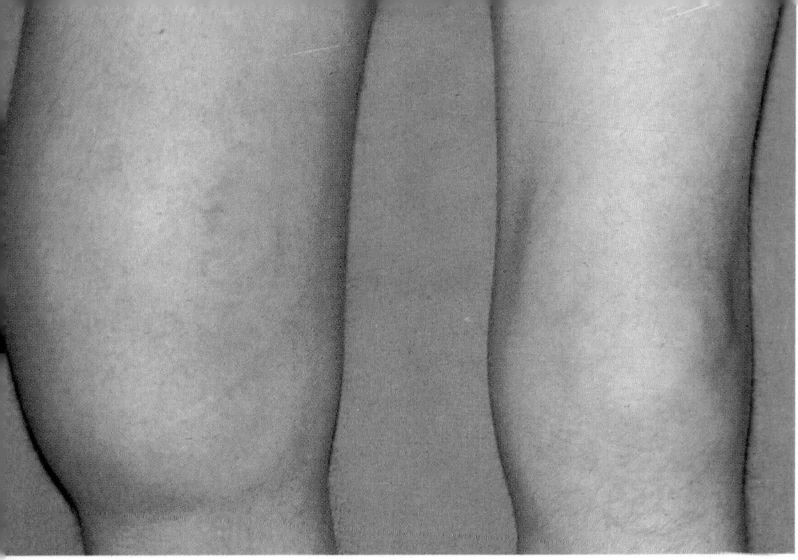

379

380

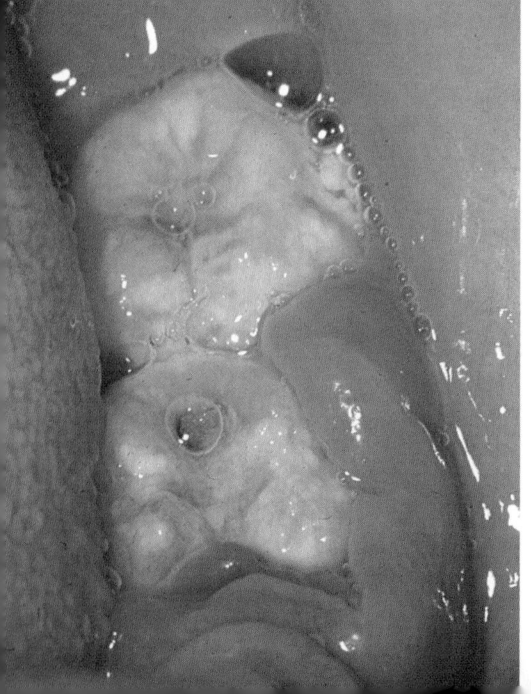

379
This teenage patient presents with an acutely swollen and painful knee after a friendly game of football.

a Why might he be at risk of developing the acquired immune deficiency syndrome?
b Which other groups are said to be at higher than normal risk?

380

a What abnormality is seen in this female patient's mouth?
b Which three causes would you consider?

381 This condition is drug-induced.
Which drugs may have been responsible?

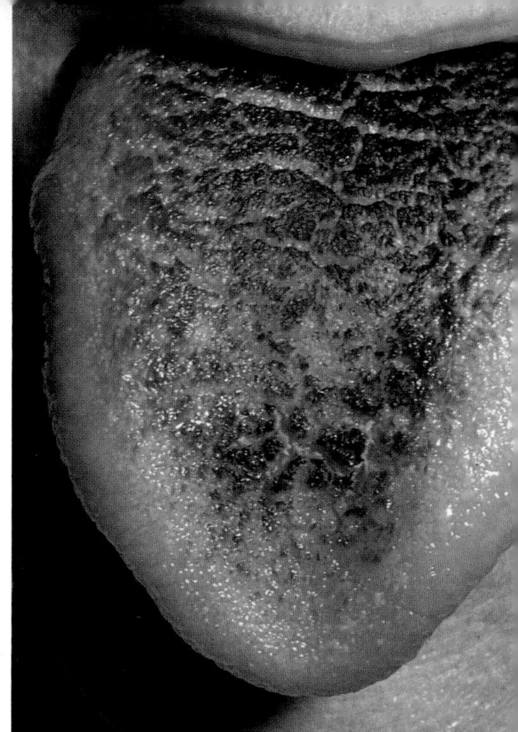

382 a What is the diagnosis?
b What abnormalities are demonstrated?

381

382

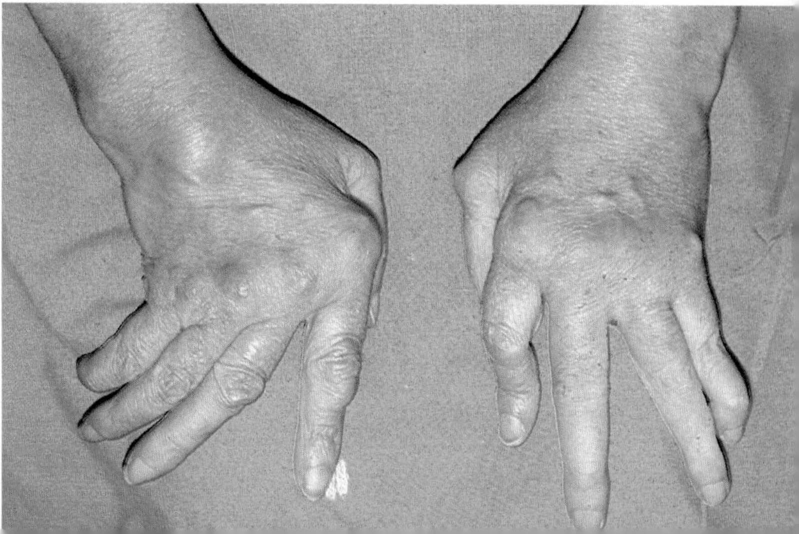

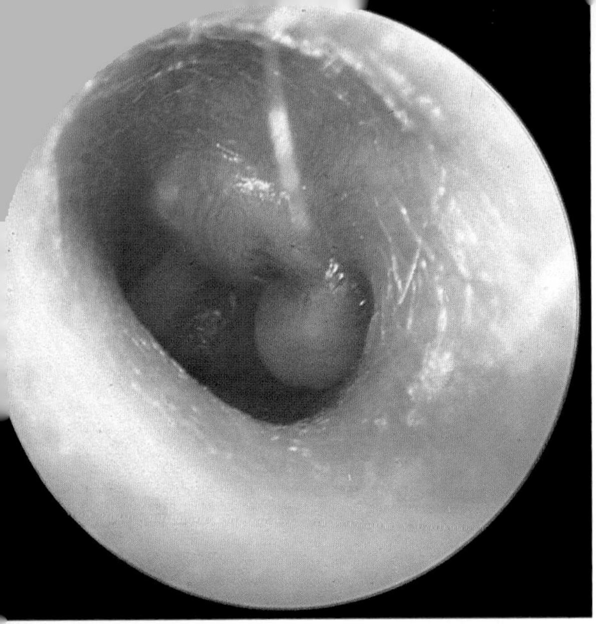

383

383 and 384

This twenty-two year old woman complained of a cough, fever and painful ear. Chest x-ray showed widespread patchy pulmonary infiltrates.

a What abnormality is shown
  i) in the blood film?
  ii) in the ear?
b What is the most likely diagnosis?
c What is the cause of the abnormality seen in the blood film?

384

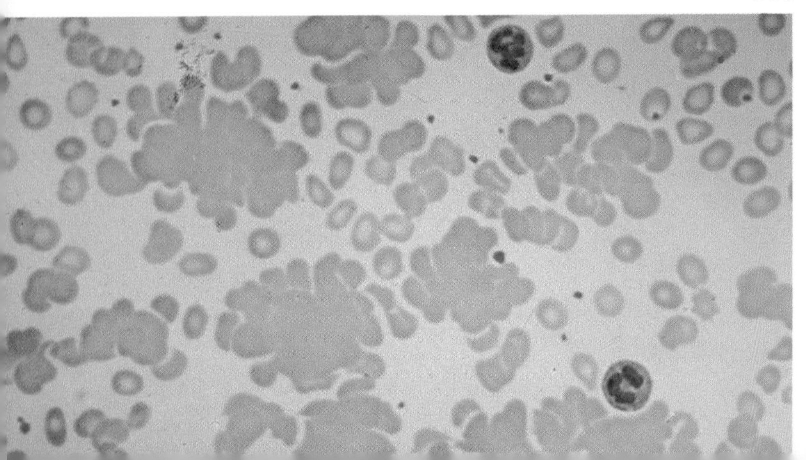

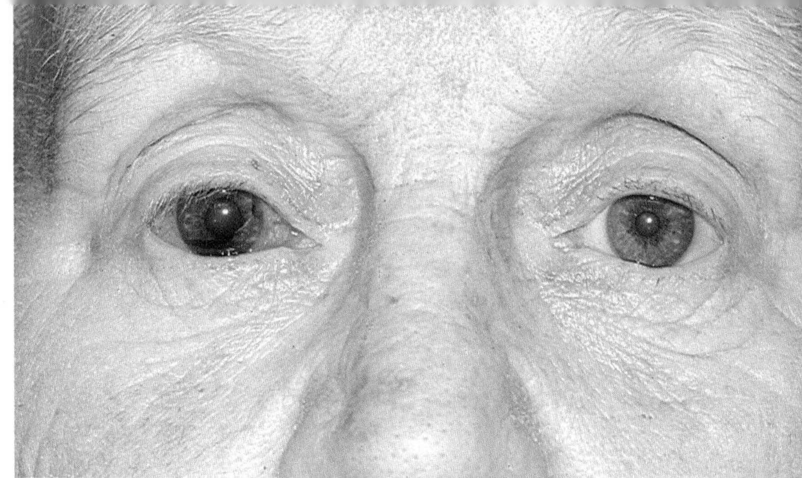

385 **385**

This woman complained of a red eye and blurred vision. There was no history of trauma.

386

a List four abnormalities present in the right eye.
b Which diagnosis does this appearance suggest?

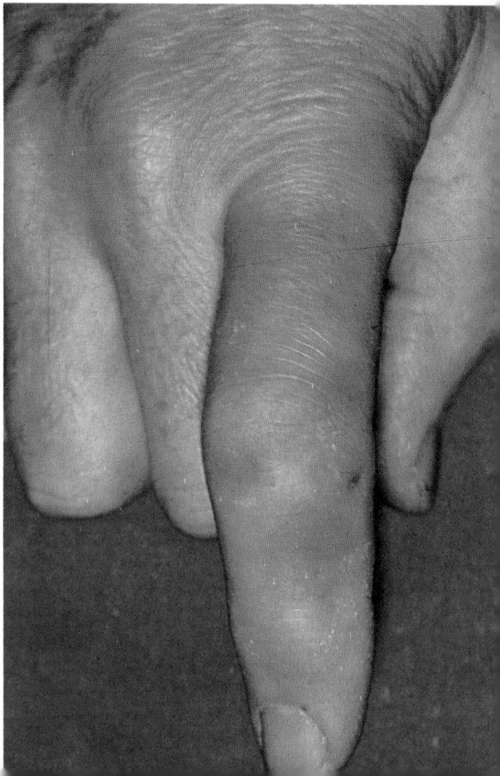

386

This man complains of a painful forefinger of several days duration. He denies any history of trauma.

a What is the likely diagnosis?
b Which occupational factors may be involved?
c What is the appropriate treatment?

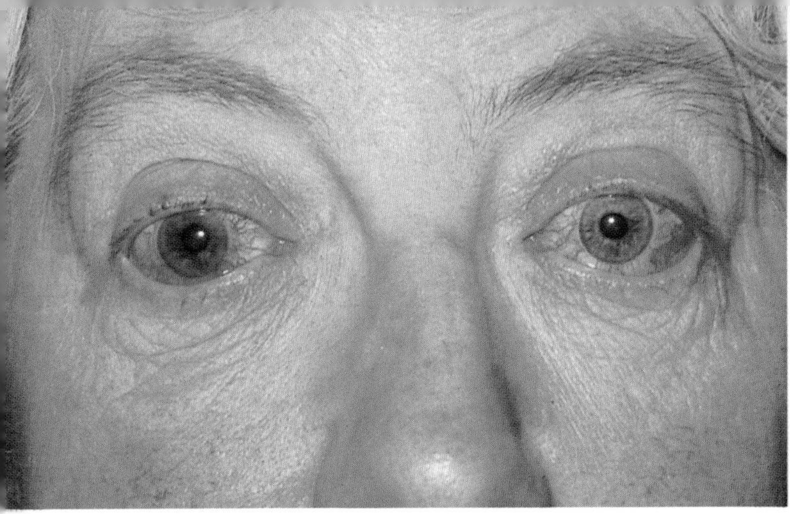

387

387 This woman complains of a roaring noise inside her head.
a What abnormalities are present?
b What is the diagnosis?
c What are the causes of this condition?

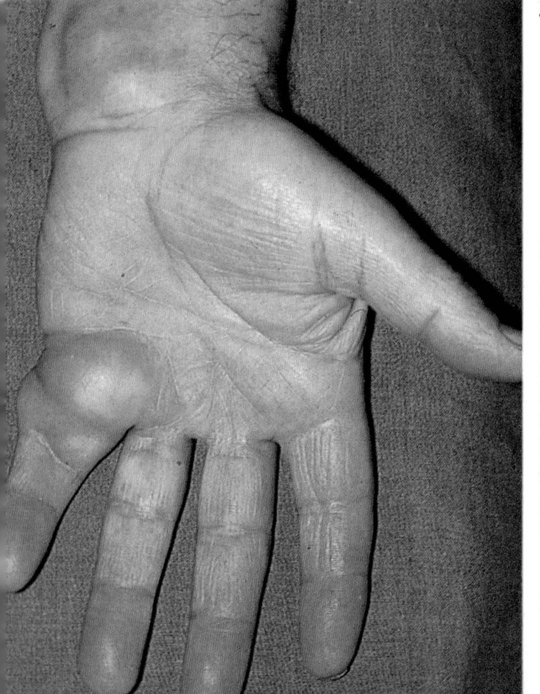

388

388
This patient has chronic renal failure. He has recently been found to have an early diastolic murmur audible along the left sternal border. His serum calcium is at the upper limit of normal; serum phosphate is greatly elevated.
a What is the most likely nature of the hand abnormality seen?
b How might this relate to his new murmur?

ANSWERS

The answers given below are necessarily brief as the aim of the series is to stimulate self-learning through further reading.

195 and 196

a Subungual fibroma.
b Phakoma.
c Tuberose sclerosis.
d 1 in 2 (usually autosomal dominant inheritance).

197 a Acromegaly.
b i) Pharmacological — bromocriptine.
ii) Irradiation — external, trans-sphenoidal implant.
iii) Surgery — transfrontal, trans-sphenoidal.
c Degree of suprasellar extension, as assessed by CT scanning.

198 a 1 — Abdominal aorta.
2 — Left adrenal tumour.
3 — Right crus of diaphragm.
4 — Top of right kidney.
5 — Tip of spleen.
b Left adrenal phaeochromocytoma. A Conn's tumour of this size is unlikely.

199 a Hyperinflation (elongated heart shadow; transverse upper ribs; anterior ends of seven ribs and posterior ends of eleven ribs visible in the lung fields).
b Acute asthma.
c Breathing in.

200 a Chronic myeloid (granulocytic) leukaemia.
b i) Cytogenetic analysis for Philadelphia chromosome.
ii) Neutrophil alkaline phosphatase score (always low).
iii) Vitamin B12 and B12 binding protein (characteristically elevated).
c i) Busulphan.
ii) Allopurinol.
iii) 6-mercaptopurine.
iv) Thioguanine.
v) Hydroxyurea.
vi) Dibromomannitol.

201 a Progressive scarring with symblepharon formation leads to loss of vision in one third of sufferers.
b Deposition of IgG, IgA, and complement at the dermo-epidermal junction.
c No.

202 a Acute inferior myocardial infarction.
b Never. In the United Kingdom, his heavy goods vehicle licence will be revoked.

203 a Ectopic ACTH secretion from a carcinoma resulting in Cushing's syndrome.
b Oat cell carcinoma of bronchus most commonly. Other sites include thymus, pancreas, and thyroid. Bronchial carcinoid tumours may secrete ACTH.
c Hypokalaemic alkalosis.
d Plasma cortisol and ACTH are usually markedly elevated and show no suppression by dexamethasone nor metyrapone. Plain chest x-ray may show bronchial carcinoma or carcinoid. CT scanning may reveal smaller tumours in the thorax or abdomen.

204 a Femoral arterial embolism.
b Left atrium.
c Atrial fibrillation (although systemic embolisation in these circumstances typically follows alteration in rhythm).

205 a Tibial pseudofractures (Looser zones).
b Pubic and ischial rami.
Scapulae (axillary border).
Femoral and humeral necks.
Ribs.
c Osteomalacia.

206 a Scabies.
b Most commonly found on the sides of fingers, flexor aspects of wrist, sole of the foot.
(Also, elbows, buttocks, axillae).
c i) Isolation of female *Sarcoptes Scabei* from skin burrows.
ii) Skin biopsy (only occasionally necessary).

207 a Ventricular septal defect.
b (Intermittent) shunt reversal (right to left).
c i) Right and left ventricular pressures approximately equal.
ii) Pulmonary artery and aortic systolic pressures equal.
iii) Pulmonary artery diastolic pressure raised (but less than aortic diastolic).
iv) Minimal or absent step-up in oxygen saturation at ventricular level.

208 a Dermatitis herpetiformis.
b Gluten-sensitive enteropathy.
c i) Gluten free diet (skin lesions may occasionally remit on this alone).
ii) Dapsone.

209 a Sycosis barbae
(a deep folliculitis of the beard area).
b Staphylococcus aureus.
c The patient's own nose.

210 a Leukoplakia.
b A pre-malignant condition.

211 a Failure of abduction of left eye.
b Left abducens (VIth) nerve palsy.

212 a i) Cullen's sign (discolouration around the umbilicus).
ii) Grey Turner's sign (flank discolouration).
b i) Leaking aortic aneurysm.
ii) Acute pancreatitis.

213 a i) Dupuytren's contractures.
ii) Palmar erythema.
b Alcoholic liver disease.
c i) White nails.
ii) Finger clubbing (more typically seen in primary biliary cirrhosis).
iii) Spider naevi.
iv) Jaundice.
v) Tremor (of alcohol withdrawal, and of hepatic failure).

214 Retinal tear with retinal detachment.

215 a Apparent hypertrophy of the calf muscles.
b Duchenne muscular dystrophy is most likely; Becker-type muscular dystrophy (also X-linked, but less severe) and myotonia congenita (rare) are also possible diagnoses.
c Gower's sign.

216 and 217
a i) Alopecia totalis, facial telangiectasia.
ii) Cutaneous calcification, resorption of distal phalanges.
b C.R.(E).S.T. syndrome. (Calcinosis, Raynaud's, (Esophageal dysmotility), Scleroderma, Telangiectasia).

218 a Ring forms of Plasmodium falciparum in erythrocytes.
b Quinine intravenously or orally depending on the clinical status of the patient.
c A combination preparation such as pyrimethamine with dapsone, or pyrimethamine with sulfadoxine.

219 a i) Spina bifida.
ii) Bilateral hydroureter and hydronephrosis.
iii) Ileal conduit (with ileostomy).
iv) Congenital dislocation of the left hip.
b Hyperchloraemia; bicarbonate depletion.
c No.

220 a Chronic lymphocytic leukaemia.
b i) Haemolytic anaemia.
ii) Hepatic infiltration.
iii) Biliary duct obstruction secondary to lymphadenopathy at the porta hepatis.
c There is an initial rise before the count falls.

221 a Pinguecula.
b None. Surgery may be considered if there is marked disfigurement.

222 and 223
a Diffuse reticulonodular shadowing, consistent with interstitial lung disease.
b Single lytic lesion, with scalloped edge and no sclerotic reaction.
c Eosinophilic granuloma (histiocytosis X).

224 a Dermatitis artefacta (cigarette burns).
b Any part of the body accessible to the hands (typically face, and non-dominant hand and arm).

225 a Olecranon bursa.
b i) Demonstration of fluctuation.
ii) Transillumination.

226 and 227
a i) Sparseness of haustral markings through most of the colon.
ii) Narrowing of the distal sigmoid.
iii) Ulceration.
iv) Pseudopolyps.
v) Loss of mucosal pattern.
b Ulcerative colitis.
c Pyoderma gangrenosum.
d i) Crohn's disease.
ii) Rheumatoid arthritis (and some other arthritides, including Behçet's disease).
iii) Myeloma/other monoclonal gammopathies.

228 and 229
a Bacterial endocarditis.
b The patient's own gastrointestinal tract.
c It is exquisitely sensitive to penicillin unlike most enteral streptococci
d There is an increased incidence of colonic carcinoma in streptococcus bovis endocarditis.

230 a Kaposi's varicelliform eruption (eczema herpeticum or vaccinatum).
b Vaccinia or herpes simplex virus.
c Pre-existing skin disease, most commonly atopic eczema. Occasionally other inflammatory dermatoses may be responsible.

231 a Widespread cellulitis of the calf; ulceration superior to the medial malleolus; ascending lymphangitis.
b Streptococcus pyogenes.
c Stasis ulceration at the ankle allowing a portal of entry.

232 Fat embolism, following femoral shaft fracture.

233 a Winged left scapula.
b Serratus anterior.
c Long thoracic nerve palsy: in this case secondary to brachial plexus involvement by apical lung tumour. (Long thoracic nerve arises from 5th, 6th and 7th cervical roots).

234 a Relapsing polychondritis.
b i) Sparing of non-cartilaginous tissue eg. lobules of the ear.
ii) Increased urinary mucopolysaccharide excretion during exacerbations.
c i) Aortitis with aortic regurgitation.
ii) Laxity of epiglottis, tracheal and bronchial rings.

235 a Blue line (Burton's line) on gums.
b Chronic lead poisoning.
c i) Anaemia.
ii) Peripheral motor neuropathy.
iii) Encephalopathy.
iv) Arthritis ('saturnine gout').

236 a Hypothyroidism.
b Thyroxine replacement.

237 Laser burns.

238 and 239
a Behçet's disease.
b The eye usually completes the triad but the joints, central nervous system, colon, skin and vascular tree may be involved.
c None.
d Men.

240 a Risus sardonicus.
b Tetanus.
c i) Phenothiazines.
ii) Metoclopramide.

241 a Gouty tophi.
b i) Serum uric acid.
ii) Compensated polarised light microscopy of expressed tophaceous material, (or of joint aspirate during an acute episode).

242 a Panhypopituitarism — craniopharyngioma.
pituitary tumour.
b i) Skull x-ray.
ii) Computed tomography head scan.
iii) Insulin hypoglycaemia — measure adrenocorticotrophic hormone, growth hormone and cortisol response.
iv) Thyrotrophin stimulation test — thyroid stimulating hormone and prolactin response.
v) Gonadotrophin stimulation tests — response of luteinising hormone and follicle stimulating hormone to gonadotrophin releasing hormone stimulation.

243 a Erythema nodosum.
b i) Sarcoidosis.
ii) Reactive arthritis.
eg. following gut infection with yersinia (pasteurella), salmonella, campylobacter jejunae.
iii) Other enteropathic arthritis — in association with inflammatory bowel disease (Crohn's, ulcerative colitis).
iv) Rheumatic fever.
v) Other uncommon possibilities include tuberculosis, polyarteritis nodosa, lepromatous leprosy, coccidioidomycosis.

244 and 245
a Keratitis (interstitial).
b Opaque material (injected bismuth) projected over both iliac crests.
c Congenital syphilis.

246 a Disseminated choroiditis. (The pigmentation is racial).
b i) Syphilis (congenital or acquired).
ii) Tuberculosis.

247 a Norwegian scabies.
b Sarcoptes scabiei hominis (— the same mite causes common human scabies. In Norwegian scabies the host response is impaired or modified).
c i) Mental deficiency.
ii) Immunodeficiency (including immunosuppressive drug therapy).
iii) Diabetes mellitus.

248 and 249
a i) Swelling right thigh (with 'bowed' appearance).
ii) Venous distension right thigh.
iii) Muscle wasting left thigh.

iv) Biopsy scar right thigh.

b i) Thickening and disordered bone formation typical of Paget's disease.

ii) Periosteal elevation with 'sun-ray' spiculation.

c Paget's disease.

d Osteosarcomatous change.

250 a Vitiligo.

b i) Diabetes mellitus.

ii) Autoimmune thyroid disease — thyroiditis, "idiopathic" hypothyroidism, Graves' disease, — also to less extent non-toxic goitre and thyroid carcinoma.

iii) Addison's disease.

iv) Other less common endocrine disorders — idiopathic hypopituitarism, autoimmune hypoparathyroidism.

251 a Symmetrical tongue enlargement.

b Acromegaly.

252 and 253

a i) Low hairline.

ii) Soft tissue swelling (in fact, lymphoedema).

b Turner's syndrome (45XO).

254 a No; the configuration of the chest leads establishes this to be true dextrocardia.

b Kartagener's syndrome.

c Chronic sinusitis; infertility.

255 a It is uncommon in women.

b Pigmentation is predominantly due to melanin deposition in the dermis.

c It is HLA linked; the HLA type varies in different affected families though breeds true within affected families.

d i) Carbohydrate tolerance improves.

ii) Cardiac failure is ameliorated.

iii) The risk of hepatoma is unchanged unless venesection is commenced before cirrhosis has begun to develop.

256 a Periventricular calcification.

b Epiloia (tuberose sclerosis).

c Rhabdomyoma.

257 a Retinitis pigmentosa.

b Abetalipoproteinaemia.

c Sensory ataxia due to posterior column degeneration is the commonest symptom. Other symptoms include muscular weakness, night blindness and ocular paresis.

d Alpha-tocopherol (vitamin E) may prevent or significantly retard the onset of neuropathy.

258 a i) Widespread nodular opacities in both lung fields.
ii) Trachea deviated to the right by neck mass.
b Thyroid carcinoma with lung metastases.

259 and 260
i) Pustular psoriasis (with psoriatic arthropathy).
ii) Reiter's syndrome.

261 a i) Failure of abduction of right eye — right VIth cranial nerve palsy.
ii) Dilated right pupil — suggesting right IIIrd cranial nerve palsy.
b i) Head or maxillofacial injury: direct nerve damage (rather than secondary to rising intracranial pressure, since the patient is fully conscious).
ii) Neurosurgery with pre-existing cranial nerve damage (eg lesion in the region of the cavernous sinus).
iii) Neurosurgery with cranial nerve damage at operation.

262 Down's syndrome (trisomy 21).

263 Acute rheumatic carditis (Carey-Coombs mitral murmur). The rash is of erythema marginatum, most typically seen on the trunk.

264 a Hidradenitis suppuritiva.
b None — no organism is consistently isolated.

265 a Sinus tachycardia; P pulmonale; right axis deviation; right ventricular hypertrophy.
b Cor pulmonale.

266 a i) Trisomy 21.
ii) Mongol mosaicism (46, XY/47, XY, + 21).
b i) Non-dysjunction.
ii) 'De novo' translocation.
iii) Familial translocation.

267 a Intracranial calcification — in curvilinear paired parallel lines.
b Sturge Weber syndrome.
c Other causes of calcification in this area include
i) Tuberose sclerosis.
ii) Congenital toxoplasmosis, cytomegalovirus infection.
iii) Angioma.
iv) Glioma (oligodendroglioma, astrocytoma).
v) Old haematoma.

268, 269 and 270
a i) Proptosis, conjunctival injection.
ii) Finger clubbing.
iii) 'Pretibial' myxoedema (in this case, in post tibial distribution).
b Graves' (or von Basedow's) disease.

271 a Discoid lupus erythematosus.
b Erythema, scaling, follicular plugging, healing with atrophy, loss of pigment, telangiectasia and scarring.
c About 5%.

272 a External angular dermoid.
b It is a congenital lesion due to inclusion of ectodermal elements at sites of ectodermal fusion.
c In all four quadrants of the orbit. In descending order of frequency: upper outer, upper inner, lower inner, lower outer.

273 a Pulmonary oedema.
b Rupture of the anterior papillary muscle causing acute mitral regurgitation or perforation of the interventricular septum.

274 a A superficial papillomatous tumour of the soft palate.
b Squamous carcinoma.
c Tobacco smoking or chewing; heavy alcohol consumption; severe iron deficiency anaemia especially in women; syphilis.

275, 276, 277 and 278
Patient 1 — Dermatitis herpetiformis.
Patient 2 — Pemphigoid.
Patient 3 — Epidermolysis bullosa (dominant dystrophic form).
Patient 4 — Pemphigus vulgaris.

279 and 280
a i) Toxic shock syndrome (TSS).
ii) Toxic epidermal necrolysis (TEN).
b Exotoxin producing staphylococci.
c The toxins have different actions. They are produced by staphylococci of differing phage type.

281 a Myasthenia gravis.
b Edrophonium chloride (Tensilon) test.
c i) CT scanning of upper mediastinum (for thymoma).
ii) Tests for associated autoimmune or connective tissue diseases. (e.g. systemic lupus erythematosus).
iii) Antibodies to acetyl choline receptor, striated muscle.
iv) Electromyography (± combined with Tensilon test).

282 a i) Pale, cloudy retina.
ii) 'Cherry red' macula.
iii) Fragmented arterial blood columns ('trucking') — seen in inferior nasal artery and branch of superior temporal artery.
b Central retinal artery occlusion.
c Yes.
d Giant cell arteritis (cranial, temporal arteritis) — tongue and jaw claudication are said to be pathognomonic of this.

283 and 284

a Xanthelasmata.
b Carotene (her sclerae are white, therefore jaundice is unlikely).
c i) Hypothyroidism.
ii) Diabetes mellitus.
iii) Familial hypercholesterolaemia.
iv) Primary biliary cirrhosis.
v) Nephrotic syndrome.

285 a No. It shows a bulky uterus.
b A Gestation sac of approximately 6 weeks.
B Intrauterine contraceptive device.

286 a i) Umbilical hernia.
ii) Gynaecomastia.
b 120 mls.
The 'Puddle Sign'. With the patient on "all fours" simultaneous percussion in the flank and auscultation around the most dependent part of the abdomen is carried out.
The presence of shifting dullness in the supine position generally indicates a litre or more of ascites. Demonstration of a fluid thrill is less sensitive.

287 a Periorbital oedema.
b Anthrax.
c Differential diagnosis includes staphylococcal infection, cow-pox, accidental vaccinia, cat scratch disease. Rarer causes include blastomycosis, sporotrichosis.
d Yes. Untreated mortality may be as high as 20%

288 a Diffuse gastric mucosal irregularity.
b 'Leather bottle stomach'; linitis plastica (diffuse adenocarcinoma).

290 a Tinea cruris due to Trichophyton rubrum.
b A topical antifungal such as miconazole, clotrimazole, or Whitfield's ointment, or systemic antifungal therapy with ketoconazole or griseofulvin.

289 a Blue rubber bleb naevus syndrome.
b Haemangiomata of bowel (usually small intestinal).
c Liver, spleen, central nervous system.

291 a i) Multiple neurofibromata.
ii) Café-au-lait spots.
b Von Recklinghausen's disease (neurofibromatosis).
c Left acoustic neuroma.

292 a Lesch-Nyhan syndrome.
b X-linked recessive.
c Hypoxanthine-guanine phosphoribosyl transferase.

293 a Caput medusae.
b Portal venous hypertension.
c i) Oesophageal varices.
ii) Acute gastric erosions.
iii) Peptic ulceration.

294 and 295
a Lid lag (Von Graeve's sign).
b It is a useful sign of thyrotoxicosis (but can also be seen in marked anxiety and with sympathomimetic drug therapy).

296 and 297
a i) Subperiosteal resorption of the phalanges, and erosion of the terminal tufts.
ii) Scratch marks.
b These suggest pre-existing chronic renal impairment (ie. acute-on-chronic uraemia).
c 1.010.

298 and 299
a Psoriatic arthropathy.
b Chloroquine or hydroxychloroquine.

300 a Absent clavicles.
b Cranio cleido dysostosis.
c i) Skull.
ii) Pubic symphysis.

301 a Clitoral hypertrophy.
b Indicates significant increase in circulating androgens.

302 a Addison's disease.
b Demonstration of an impaired cortisol response to 250 μg aqueous tetracosactrin given intramuscularly.
c Eosinophilia; lymphocytosis.

303 a Neovascularisation.
b Diabetes mellitus and sickle cell disease are the commonest causes. Others include hyperviscosity syndromes; sarcoidosis; Behçet's disease; Eales disease; exudative retinopathy.

304 No. The lack of skin creases indicates that it is less than thirty-six weeks gestation.

305 a Rupture of the long head of biceps.
b There is usually no significant loss of power.
c Repeated local injections of corticosteroids for bicipital tendonitis.

306 and 307

a i) Left pleural effusion.
  ii) Left pneumothorax.
  iii) Mediastinal shift to the left.
  iv) Surgical clips left upper zone (on stump of left upper lobe bronchus).
  v) Pleural fluid/thickening right cardiophrenic angle.

b Widespread nodular opacities in both lung fields.

c Bronchial carcinoma with pulmonary metastases.
(The upper film was taken shortly after thoracotomy for left upper lobectomy).

308 i) Her 'normal' serum thyroxine (T4) may have been at the low end of the normal range. 148 nmol/l may therefore represent as much as a two-fold rise.
  ii) Isolated T3 (tri-iodothyronine) toxicosis.
  iii) Diminished concentration of thyroxine binding globulin (TBG). This may represent a normal variant; or may be secondary to thyrotoxicosis itself, nephrotic syndrome, or to an inherited, sex-linked deficiency in TBG. Drug-induced reduction in TBG (eg high dose corticosteroids, testosterone) is unlikely here, as is active acromegaly.
  iv) Displacement of T4 from TBG, increased degradation of T4 (both may occur with phenytoin therapy).
  v) Euthyroidism — the clinical features may be those of anxiety.
  vi) Sampling or laboratory error.

309 1 True aortic lumen.
2 False aortic lumen.
3 Intimal flap of dissection.
4 Right kidney with white cortex and darker medulla.
5 Tip of right lobe of liver.

310 a Yes.
b This is a kerion due to cattle ringworm, Trichophyton verrucosum.
c Oral antifungal therapy (griseofulvin or ketoconazole) plus systemic antibiotic to eradicate bacterial superinfection.

311 i) Mycobacterium tuberculosis.
  ii) Staphylococcus aureus.
  iii) Klebsiella pneumoniae.
  iv) Bacteroides (and other anaerobes).
  v) Others include:
  Actinomycosis, histoplasmosis, coccidioidomycosis, aspergillosis, nocardiosis.

312 a Leptospirosis (Weil's disease).
b Yes. Leptospirosis was formerly common in this group.
c Rodents, particularly the brown rat in the United Kingdom.

313 a Cutaneous larva migrans (creeping eruption).
b Ancylostoma brasiliense is the commonest cause but others include A. caninum, Strongyloides stercoralis, Necator americanus, and Gasterophilus.

314 VIIth nerve neuroma in association with neurofibromatosis. Pigmented 'café au lait' patches are seen on the trunk (in addition to an old biopsy scar in the neck).

315 a Acromegaly.
b Median nerve compression (carpal tunnel syndrome).

316 a High myopic degeneration.
b Long.

317 a Secondary syphilis.
b Diffuse proliferative glomerulonephritis.

318 i) Enlargement, erosion, and/or double floor of the pituitary fossa.
ii) Enlargement of the frontal sinuses.
iii) Increase in the angle of the mandible.
iv) Prognathism.
v) Thickening of the cranial vault.

319 a Scurvy (Vitamin C deficiency).
b No.
c i) Platelet ascorbic acid levels (plasma levels less helpful).
ii) Ascorbic acid saturation test.

320 and 321
a i) Distended superficial veins. (The right chest has also been recently shaved, and radiotherapy markers are visible).
ii) Large irregular opacity in the right upper zone; enlargement of right hilum and upper mediastinum.
b Superior vena caval obstruction, secondary to bronchogenic carcinoma with massive mediastinal lymphadenopathy.
c Radiotherapy.

322 a Fissuring of the lateral margins of the tongue.
b Recurrent facial palsy.
c Melkersson's syndrome.

323 a Air in the soft tissues.
b Gas gangrene. (Infection with gas-forming organisms, eg clostridium perfringens).

324 a Osteogenesis imperfecta congenita (in this form, type III osteogenesis imperfecta, the sclerae are often white).
b Hyperplastic callus formation (possibly in relation to fracture; not necessarily so).

325 a Benign melanoma of the choroid.
b None, but the patient should be followed up with regular fundal photographs.

326 a Fixed drug eruption.
b i) Tetracycline.
ii) Sulphonamide (eg sulphamethoxazole, as in co-trimoxazole).
c Oral challenge — lesion, once healed, will reappear two to three hours after ingestion of the offending drug. This does not carry a risk of anaphylaxis.
(patch tests on involved skin give variable results; on uninvolved skin, patch testing is negative).

327 The ECG should be repeated at the correct voltage. It proves to be completely normal.

328 a Nodular prurigo.
b None. Local infiltration with corticosteroid may be helpful, usually briefly.

329 a Hydatid disease (Echinococcosis).
b Global.
c Man is an accidental intermediate host.

330 a Oral candidiasis (thrush).
b Broad-spectrum antibiotics; corticosteroids; immunosuppressive agents.

331 a Lumbar myelogram (using water-soluble contrast medium).
b Lateral protrusion of the L5/S1 disc (right side).
c i) Impaired sensation on the outer border of foot (including fourth and fifth toes) and sole (sparing the great toe).
ii) Weakness is usually limited to the toe dorsiflexors (especially extensor hallucis longus).
iii) Impaired or absent ankle jerk.

332 a Basal cell carcinoma (rodent ulcer).
b No —
i) Dissemination of basal cell carcinoma is uncommon (lymphatic dissemination more so).
ii) Lymphatic drainage from post-auricular skin is not to the submandibular nodes (rather, to retroauricular and upper deep cervical nodes).

333 and 334
a i) Hyperextensible joints.
ii) 'Papyraceous' scar.
b Ehlers Danlos syndrome.
c Mitral valve prolapse ('floppy' mitral valve).

335 a Chloasma of pregnancy.
b Breasts, linea alba (becoming linea nigra); occasionally in striae gravidarum.

336 a Pigmentation.
b Addison's disease.
c The development of Addison's disease must have been more than two years ago.

337 and 338
a Pulmonary actinomycosis.
b None.
c The source of infection is usually the mouth. The pulmonary infection is often due to aspiration. Poor oral hygiene is more typically related to cervicofacial actinomycosis.

339 a Periorbital cellulitis.
b Non-fatal complications include,
i) Cavernous sinus thrombosis.
ii) Meningitis.
iii) Brain abscess.
iv) Optic atrophy.
c Helpful signs include,
i) Impaired visual acuity.
ii) Pupillary defects.
iii) Papilloedema.
iv) Raised intraocular pressure.

340 a Shingles (herpes zoster).
b Cervical 7 and 8.

341 a Acne rosacea.
b i) Conjunctivitis.
ii) Blepharitis.
iii) Hordeolum (stye).
iv) Keratitis.

342 a Left apical pneumothorax.

343 a Eyeball prosthesis.
b He has metastatic malignant melanoma from choroidal melanoma (the affected eye having been enucleated).

344 a Erythroderma.
b Chronic lymphatic leukaemia, Hodgkin's disease.
c i) Hypothermia.
ii) Infections — cutaneous, respiratory.
iii) Thrombophlebitis.
iv) Peripheral circulatory failure.

345 a Von Willebrand's disease.
b It will be prolonged.
c Normal aggregation to collagen.
d 50% of boys.

346 a Mycetoma (Madura foot).
b None. (Madura foot is caused by fungi and, occasionally, actinomycetes).
c None.

347 No sign will reliably differentiate between the conditions.

348 a Scrofula.
b Mycobacterium tuberculosis, though bovine or atypical mycobacteria may be causative.

349 and 350
a Paget's disease.
b Not necessarily: specific treatment is indicated if there is sensorineural impairment secondary to skull foraminal compression; more often, deafness in Paget's disease is due to involvement of the ossicles or to coincidental disease.

351 a Rheumatoid nodules.
b Fibrous stroma containing granulomatous foci. Each granuloma consists of
i) A central zone of fibrinoid necrosis, containing cellular and nuclear debris, and fibrin.
ii) A rim of fibroblasts and histiocytes arranged in palisades.
iii) A surrounding chronic inflammatory infiltrate (plasma cells, lymphocytes, occasional giant cells).
c Positive tests for rheumatoid factor (Rose Waaler, RA latex tests).

352 a Neck webbing.
b Turner's syndrome.
c Coarctation of the aorta.

353 and 354
a i) Choroiditis.
ii) Intracerebral calcification.
b Congenital toxoplasmosis.

355 a Staining of teeth due to tetracycline administration.
b Tetracycline-stained teeth may fluoresce when viewed in ultra-violet light.
c Differing rates of odontogenesis and calcification of individual teeth modify the amount of tetracycline taken up by the teeth.
d No, in fact they are less prone than normal to caries.

356 a i) Right mastectomy.
ii) Local recurrence of breast carcinoma.

iii) Oedema of the arm.
iv) Radiation skin damage.
b Cutaneous haemiangiosarcoma (Stewart-Treves syndrome).

357 a Imperforate anus; meconium issuing from the urethra.
b Rectovesical or rectourethral fistula.

358 a Embolism of mural thrombus from the left ventricle. A recent anterior myocardial infarction is seen on the ECG.
b Yes, unless there is a contraindication. There have been no adequate clinical studies to determine the optimal time to anticoagulate such patients, but delayed anticoagulation is associated with a higher incidence of recurrent embolism.
c Mural thrombus may be detected by two-dimensional echocardiography, contrast ventriculography, or radionucleide scanning.

359 a Carbuncle.
b Diabetes mellitus.

360 and 361
a Erythema multiforme.
b Organisms include herpes simplex, mycoplasma pneumoniae, chlamydiae, orf and streptococci.
c No, though they may help differentiate it from diseases such as pemphigoid if there is doubt.

362 a Prolapse of a tumour mass into the left ventricle.
b Left atrial myxoma (with systemic embolisation).
c Cardiac surgery, as soon as possible.

363 Femoral arterial blood sampling for blood gas analysis.

364 a Bilateral pitting arm oedema.
b Superior vena caval obstruction.
c Lymphoma, especially Hodgkin's.
d Massive upper mediastinal lymphadenopathy.

365 a i) Plantar erythema.
ii) Trophic ulcer.
b Alcohol — causing liver disease and peripheral sensory neuropathy. (Diabetes mellitus and vasculitic rheumatoid arthritis are less likely possibilities).

366 a Microaneurysms, dot haemorrhages and hard exudates.
b i) Urinalysis for glucose.
ii) Plasma glucose: fasting, postprandial or as part of an oral glucose tolerance test.

367 and 368

a Band keratopathy.
b Swelling of right shoulder (due to subcutaneous calcification).
c Tertiary hyperparathyroidism.

369 a 'Fresh' striae (atrophicae).
b Cushing's syndrome.
c They cannot be discriminated with certainty. Distribution, appearance and histology may be the same.

370 a None. The epiphysis of the tubercle is beginning to ossify but this appearance is normal.
b Osteochondritis of the tibial apophysis (Osgood — Schlatter's disease).
c None. Restriction of excessive physical activity or occasionally a walking long leg plaster may be suggested.

371 and 372

a Spina bifida occulta.
b Diastematomyelia — with linear growth, stretching of tethered cord and nerve roots across fibrous septum leads to nerve root damage and splitting of the cord.

373 and 374

a Arthritis mutilans.
b Rheumatoid arthritis.
c i) Periarticular soft tissue swelling.
ii) Periarticular osteoporosis.
iii) Joint space narrowing.

375, 376, 377 and 378

a Facioscapulohumeral muscular dystrophy.
b i) Weak tibialis anterior.
ii) Impaired biceps, triceps reflexes. Supinator, knee and ankle jerks normal.
c i) Orbicularis oris, serratus anterior.
ii) Left pectoralis major (which is absent).
d Life expectancy is usually normal.

379 a He is haemophiliac. A.I.D.S. may be transmissable in blood products.
b Male homosexuals and their contacts.
Heroin addicts.
Haitians.

380 a Gum hyperplasia/hypertrophy/infiltration.
b i) Phenytoin (in association with bacterial plaque).
ii) Normal pregnancy (and oral contraceptives).
iii) Acute myelomonocytic leukaemia.

381 i) Oral penicillins.
ii) Other topical oral antibiotics and mouthwashes (eg. sodium perborate).
iii) Bismuth.

382 a Rheumatoid arthritis.
b i) Ulnar deviation and prominent metacarpal heads (subluxation at MCP joints).
ii) Boutonniere (index left) and swan neck (5th left) deformities.
iii) Extensor tendon nodules.
iv) Wasting of dorsal interossei.
(This patient also has ruptured 3rd, 4th and 5th extensor tendons on the right with prominent right ulnar styloid).

383 and 384
a i) Red cell agglutination.
ii) Bullous myringitis.
b Mycoplasma pneumoniae infection.
c Cold agglutination occurs due to the development of a macroglobulin (IgM) directed against I antigen on the red cell surface.

385 a i) Hyphaema.
ii) Conjunctival suffusion.
iii) Irregular, dilated pupil.
iv) Depression of the iris at the limbus in the three o'clock position.
b The abnormalities of the iris and pupil in the absence of trauma suggest a tumour of the ciliary body, most likely a malignant melanoma. (The iris appearance should not be mistaken for an iridectomy, which is unlikely at this site).

386 a Erysipeloid due to cutaneous infection by Erysipelothrix rhusiopathiae.
b It is most commonly seen in abbatoir or fish workers.
c The organism is sensitive to penicillins, cephalosporins, erythromycin, tetracyclines, and chloramphenicol.

387 a i) Bilateral exophthalmos.
ii) Conjunctival injection.
b Carotico-cavernous fistula.
c Spontaneous rupture of an infraclinoid aneurysm into the cavernous sinus; traumatic following skull fracture (particularly basitemporal fracture) or neurosurgery.

388 a Subcutaneous calcification.
b Metastatic calcification in the aortic valve may have led to aortic incompetence.

INDEX

TABLETS

PLENDIL®

(FELODIPINE, MSD)

EXTENDED-RELEASE TABLETS

DESCRIPTION

PLENDIL* (Felodipine, MSD) is a calcium antagonist (calcium channel blocker). Felodipine is a dihydropyridine derivative that is chemically described as ± ethyl methyl 4-(2,3-dichlorophenyl)-1, 4-dihydro-2,6-dimethyl-3,5-pyridinedicarboxylate. Its empirical formula is $C_{18}H_{19}Cl_2NO_4$ and its structural formula is:

H H_3C N CH_3 H_3COOC $COOCH_2CH_3$ Cl Cl

Felodipine is a slightly yellowish, crystalline powder with a molecular weight of 384.26. It is insoluble in water and is freely soluble in dichloromethane and ethanol. Felodipine is a racemic mixture.

Tablets PLENDIL provide extended release of felodipine. They are available as tablets containing 5 mg or 10 mg of felodipine for oral administration. In addition to the active ingredient felodipine, each tablet contains the following inactive ingredients: cellulose, iron oxides, lactose, polyethylene glycol, sodium stearyl fumarate, titanium dioxide and other ingredients.

CLINICAL PHARMACOLOGY

Mechanism of Action

Felodipine is a member of the dihydropyridine class of calcium channel antagonists (calcium channel blockers). It reversibly competes with nitrendipine and/or other calcium channel blockers for dihydropyridine binding sites, blocks voltage-dependent Ca^{++} currents in vascular smooth muscle and cultured rabbit atrial cells and blocks potassium-induced contracture of the rat portal vein.

In vitro studies show that the effects of felodipine on contractile processes are selective, with greater effects on vascular smooth muscle than cardiac muscle. Negative inotropic effects can be detected *in vitro*, but such effects have not been seen in intact animals.

The effect of felodipine on blood pressure is principally a consequence of a dose-related decrease of peripheral vascular resistance in man, with a modest reflex increase in heart rate (see *Cardiovascular Effects*). With the exception of a mild diuretic effect seen in several animal species and man, the effects of felodipine are accounted for by its effects on peripheral vascular resistance.

Pharmacokinetics and Metabolism

Following oral administration, felodipine is almost completely absorbed and undergoes extensive first-pass metabolism. The systemic bioavailability of PLENDIL is approximately 20 percent. Mean peak concentrations following the administration of PLENDIL are reached in 2.5 to 5 hours. Both peak plasma concentration and the area under the plasma concentration time curve (AUC) increase linearly with doses up to 20 mg. Felodipine is greater than 99 percent bound to plasma proteins.

Following intravenous administration, the plasma concentration of felodipine declined triexponentially with mean disposition half-lives of 4.8 minutes, 1.5 hours and 9.1 hours. The mean contributions of the three individual phases to the overall AUC were 15, 40 and 45 percent, respectively, in the order of increasing $t_{\frac{1}{2}}$.

Following oral administration of the immediate-release formulation, the plasma level of felodipine also declined polyexponentially with a mean terminal $t_{\frac{1}{2}}$ of 11 to 16 hours. The mean peak and trough steady-state plasma concentrations achieved after 10 mg of the immediate-release formulation given once a day to normal volunteers, were 20 and 0.5 nmol/L, respectively. The trough plasma concentration of felodipine in most individuals was substantially below the concentration needed to effect a half-maximal decline in blood pressure (EC_{50}) [4-6 nmol/L for felodipine], thus precluding once a day dosing with the immediate-release formulation.

Following administration of a 10-mg dose of PLENDIL, the extended-release formulation, to young, healthy volunteers, mean peak and trough steady-state plasma concentrations of felodipine were 7 and 2 nmol/L, respectively. Corresponding values in hypertensive patients (mean age 64) after a 20-mg dose of PLENDIL were 23 and 7 nmol/L. Since the EC_{50} for felodipine is 4 to 6 nmol/L, a 5 to 10-mg dose of PLENDIL in some patients, and a 20-mg dose in others, would be expected to provide an antihypertensive effect that persists for 24 hours (see *Cardiovascular Effects* below and DOSAGE AND ADMINISTRATION).

The systemic plasma clearance of felodipine in young healthy subjects is about 0.8 L/min and the apparent volume of distribution is about 10 L/kg.

Following an oral or intravenous dose of ^{14}C-labeled felodipine in man, about 70 percent of the dose of radioactivity was recovered in urine and 10 percent in the feces. A negligible amount of intact felodipine is recovered in the urine and feces (<0.5%). Six metabolites, which account for 23 percent of the oral dose, have been identified; none has significant vasodilating activity.

Following administration of PLENDIL to hypertensive patients, mean peak plasma concentrations at steady state are about 20 percent higher than after a single dose. Blood pressure response is correlated with plasma concentrations of felodipine.

The bioavailability of PLENDIL is not influenced by the presence of food in the gastrointestinal tract. In a study of six patients, the bioavailability of felodipine was increased more than two-fold when taken with doubly concentrated grapefruit juice, compared to when taken with water or orange juice. A similar finding has been seen with some other dihydropyridine calcium antagonists, but to a lesser extent than that seen with felodipine.

Age Effects: Plasma concentrations of felodipine, after a single dose and at steady state, increase with age. Mean clearance of felodipine in elderly hypertensives (mean age 74) was only 45 percent of that of young volunteers (mean age 26). At steady state mean AUC for young patients was 39 percent of that for the elderly. Data for intermediate age ranges suggest that the AUCs fall between the extremes of the young and the elderly.

Hepatic Dysfunction: In patients with hepatic disease, the clearance of felodipine was reduced to about 60 percent of that seen in normal young volunteers.

Renal impairment does not alter the plasma concentration profile of felodipine; although higher concentrations of the metabolites are present in the plasma due to decreased urinary excretion, these are inactive.

MSD is a registered trademark of MERCK & CO., INC.
*Registered trademark of AB Astra

Animal studies have demonstrated that felodipine crosses the blood-brain barrier and the placenta.

Cardiovascular Effects

Following administration of PLENDIL, a reduction in blood pressure generally occurs within two to five hours. During chronic administration, substantial blood pressure control lasts for 24 hours, with trough reductions in diastolic blood pressure approximately 40-50 percent of peak reductions. The antihypertensive effect is dose-dependent and correlates with the plasma concentration of felodipine.

A reflex increase in heart rate frequently occurs during the first week of therapy; this increase attenuates over time. Heart rate increases of 5-10 beats per minute may be seen during chronic dosing. The increase is inhibited by beta-blocking agents.

The P-R interval of the ECG is not affected by felodipine when administered alone or in combination with a beta-blocking agent. Felodipine alone or in combination with a beta-blocking agent has been shown, in clinical and electrophysiologic studies, to have no significant effect on cardiac conduction (P-R, P-Q and H-V intervals).

In clinical trials in hypertensive patients without clinical evidence of left ventricular dysfunction, no symptoms suggestive of a negative inotropic effect were noted; however none would be expected in this population (see PRECAUTIONS).

Renal/Endocrine Effects

Renal vascular resistance is decreased by felodipine while glomerular filtration rate remains unchanged. Mild diuresis, natriuresis and kaliuresis have been observed during the first week of therapy. No significant effects on serum electrolytes were observed during short- and long-term therapy.

In clinical trials increases in plasma noradrenaline levels have been observed.

Clinical Studies

Felodipine produces dose-related decreases in systolic and diastolic blood pressure as demonstrated in six placebo-controlled, dose response studies using either immediate-release or extended-release dosage forms. These studies enrolled over 800 patients on active treatment, at total daily doses ranging from 2.5 to 20 mg. In those studies felodipine was administered either as monotherapy or was added to beta blockers. The results of the two studies with PLENDIL given once daily as monotherapy are shown in the table below:

MEAN REDUCTIONS IN BLOOD PRESSURE (mmHg)*
Systolic/Diastolic

Dose	N	Mean Peak Response	Mean Trough Response	Trough/Peak Ratios (%s)
Study 1 (8 weeks)				
2.5 mg	68	9.4/4.7	2.7/2.5	29/53
5 mg	69	9.5/6.3	2.4/3.7	25/59
10 mg	67	18.0/10.8	10.0/6.0	56/56
Study 2 (4 weeks)				
10 mg	50	5.3/7.2	1.5/3.2	33/40**
20 mg	50	11.3/10.2	4.5/3.2	43/34**

*Placebo response subtracted

**Different number of patients available for peak and trough measurements

INDICATIONS AND USAGE

PLENDIL is indicated for the treatment of hypertension. PLENDIL may be used alone or concomitantly with other antihypertensive agents.

CONTRAINDICATIONS

PLENDIL is contraindicated in patients who are hypersensitive to this product.

PLENDIL®
(Felodipine, MSD)
Extended-Release Tablets

PRECAUTIONS

General

Hypotension: Felodipine, like other calcium antagonists, may occasionally precipitate significant hypotension and rarely syncope. It may lead to reflex tachycardia which in susceptible individuals may precipitate angina pectoris. (See ADVERSE REACTIONS.)

Heart Failure: Although acute hemodynamic studies in a small number of patients with NYHA Class II or III heart failure treated with felodipine have not demonstrated negative inotropic effects, safety in patients with heart failure has not been established. Caution therefore should be exercised when using PLENDIL in patients with heart failure or compromised ventricular function, particularly in combination with a beta blocker.

Elderly Patients or Patients with Impaired Liver Function: Patients over 65 years of age or patients with impaired liver function may have elevated plasma concentrations of felodipine and may therefore respond to lower doses of PLENDIL. These patients should have their blood pressure monitored closely during dosage adjustment of PLENDIL and should rarely require doses above 10 mg. (See CLINICAL PHARMACOLOGY and DOSAGE AND ADMINISTRATION.)

Peripheral Edema: Peripheral edema, generally mild and not associated with generalized fluid retention, was the most common adverse event in the clinical trials. The incidence of peripheral edema was both dose- and age-dependent. Frequency of peripheral edema ranged from about 10 percent in patients under 50 years of age taking 5 mg daily to about 30 percent in those over 60 years of age taking 20 mg daily. This adverse effect generally occurs within 2-3 weeks of the initiation of treatment.

Information for Patients

Patients should be instructed to take PLENDIL whole and not to crush or chew the tablets. They should be told that mild gingival hyperplasia (gum swelling) has been reported. Good dental hygiene decreases its incidence and severity.

NOTE: As with many other drugs, certain advice to patients being treated with PLENDIL is warranted. This information is intended to aid in the safe and effective use of this medication. It is not a disclosure of all possible adverse or intended effects.

Drug Interactions

Beta-Blocking Agents: A pharmacokinetic study of felodipine in conjunction with metoprolol demonstrated no significant effects on the pharmacokinetics of felodipine. The AUC and C_{max} of metoprolol, however, were increased approximately 31 and 38 percent, respectively. In controlled clinical trials, however, beta blockers including metoprolol were concurrently administered with felodipine and were well tolerated.

Cimetidine: In healthy subjects pharmacokinetic studies showed an approximately 50 percent increase in the area under the plasma concentration time curve (AUC) as well as the C_{max} of felodipine when given concomitantly with cimetidine. It is anticipated that a clinically significant interaction may occur in some hypertensive patients. Therefore, it is recommended that low doses of PLENDIL be used when given concomitantly with cimetidine.

Digoxin: When given concomitantly with felodipine the peak plasma concentration of digoxin was significantly increased. There was, however, no significant change in the AUC of digoxin.

Other Concomitant Therapy: In healthy subjects there were no clinically significant interactions when felodipine was given concomitantly with indomethacin or spironolactone.

Interaction with Food: See CLINICAL PHARMACOLOGY, *Pharmacokinetics and Metabolism.*

Carcinogenesis, Mutagenesis, Impairment of Fertility

In a two-year carcinogenicity study in rats fed felodipine at doses of 7.7, 23.1 or 69.3 mg/kg/day (up to 28 times* the maximum recommended human dose on a mg/m^2 basis), a dose-related increase in the incidence of benign interstitial cell tumors of the testes (Leydig cell tumors) was observed in treated male rats. These tumors were not observed in a similar study in mice at doses up to 138.6 mg/kg/day (28 times* the maximum recommended human dose on a mg/m^2 basis). Felodipine, at the doses employed in the two-year rat study, has been shown to lower testicular testosterone and to produce a corresponding increase in serum luteinizing hormone in rats. The Leydig cell tumor development is possibly secondary to these hormonal effects which have not been observed in man.

In this same rat study a dose-related increase in the incidence of focal squamous cell hyperplasia compared to control was observed in the esophageal groove of male and female rats in all dose groups. No other drug-related esophageal or gastric pathology was observed in the rats or with chronic administration in mice and dogs. The latter species, like man, has no anatomical structure comparable to the esophageal groove.

Felodipine was not carcinogenic when fed to mice at doses of up to 138.6 mg/kg/day (28 times* the maximum recommended human dose on a mg/m^2 basis) for periods of up to 80 weeks in males and 99 weeks in females.

Felodipine did not display any mutagenic activity *in vitro* in the Ames microbial mutagenicity test or in the mouse lymphoma forward mutation assay. No clastogenic potential was seen *in vivo* in the mouse micronucleus test at oral doses up to 2500 mg/kg (506 times* the maximum recommended human dose on a mg/m^2 basis) or *in vitro* in a human lymphocyte chromosome aberration assay.

A fertility study in which male and female rats were administered doses of 3.8, 9.6 or 26.9 mg/kg/day showed no significant effect of felodipine on reproductive performance.

Pregnancy

Pregnancy Category C

Teratogenic Effects: Studies in pregnant rabbits administered doses of 0.46, 1.2, 2.3 and 4.6 mg/kg/day (from 0.4 to 4 times* the maximum recommended human dose on a mg/m^2 basis) showed digital anomalies consisting of reduction in size and degree of ossification of the terminal phalanges in the fetuses. The frequency and severity of the changes appeared dose-related and were noted even at the lowest dose. These changes have been shown to occur with other members of the dihydropyridine class and are possibly a result of compromised uterine blood flow. Similar fetal anomalies were not observed in rats given felodipine.

In a teratology study in cynomolgus monkeys no reduction in the size of the terminal phalanges was observed but an abnormal position of the distal phalanges was noted in about 40 percent of the fetuses.

Nonteratogenic Effects: A prolongation of parturition with difficult labor and an increased frequency of fetal and early postnatal deaths were observed in rats administered doses of 9.6 mg/kg/day (4 times* the maximum human dose on a mg/m^2 basis) and above.

*Based on patient weight of 50 kg

Significant enlargement of the mammary glands in excess of the normal enlargement for pregnant rabbits was found with doses greater than or equal to 1.2 mg/kg/day (equal to the maximum human dose on a mg/m^2 basis). This effect occurred only in pregnant rabbits and regressed during lactation. Similar changes in the mammary glands were not observed in rats or monkeys.

There are no adequate and well-controlled studies in pregnant women. If felodipine is used during pregnancy, or if the patient becomes pregnant while taking this drug, she should be apprised of the potential hazard to the fetus, possible digital anomalies of the infant, and the potential effects of felodipine on labor and delivery, and on the mammary glands of pregnant females.

Nursing Mothers

It is not known whether this drug is secreted in human milk and because of the potential for serious adverse reactions from felodipine in the infant, a decision should be made whether to discontinue nursing or to discontinue the drug, taking into account the importance of the drug to the mother.

Pediatric Use

Safety and effectiveness in children have not been established.

ADVERSE REACTIONS

In controlled studies in the United States and overseas approximately 3000 patients were treated with felodipine as either the extended-release or the immediate-release formulation.

The most common clinical adverse experiences reported with PLENDIL administered as monotherapy in all settings and with all dosage forms of felodipine were peripheral edema and headache. Peripheral edema was generally mild, but it was age- and dose-related and resulted in discontinuation of therapy in about 4 percent of the enrolled patients. Discontinuation of therapy due to any clinical adverse experience occurred in about 9 percent of the patients receiving PLENDIL, principally for peripheral edema, headache, or flushing.

Adverse experiences that occurred with an incidence of 1.5 percent or greater during monotherapy with PLENDIL without regard to causality are compared to placebo in the table below.

Percent of Patients with Adverse Effects in Controlled Trials of PLENDIL as Monotherapy
(Incidence of discontinuations shown in parentheses)

Adverse Effect	PLENDIL % N = 730		Placebo % N = 283
Peripheral Edema	22.3	(4.2)	3.5
Headache	18.6	(2.1)	10.6
Flushing	6.4	(1.0)	1.1
Dizziness	5.8	(0.8)	3.2
Upper Respiratory Infection	5.5	(0.1)	1.1
Asthenia	4.7	(0.1)	2.8
Cough	2.9	(0.0)	0.4
Paresthesia	2.5	(0.1)	1.8
Dyspepsia	2.3	(0.0)	1.4
Chest Pain	2.1	(0.1)	1.4
Nausea	1.9	(0.8)	1.1
Muscle Cramps	1.9	(0.0)	1.1
Palpitation	1.8	(0.5)	2.5
Abdominal Pain	1.8	(0.3)	1.1
Constipation	1.6	(0.1)	1.1
Diarrhea	1.6	(0.1)	1.1
Pharyngitis	1.6	(0.0)	0.4
Rhinorrhea	1.6	(0.0)	0.0
Back Pain	1.6	(0.0)	1.1
Rash	1.5	(0.1)	1.1

*Based on patient weight of 50 kg

In the two dose response studies using PLENDIL as monotherapy, the following table describes the incidence (percent) of adverse experiences that were dose-related:

Adverse Effect	Placebo N = 121	2.5 mg N = 71	5.0 mg N = 72	10.0 mg N = 123	20 mg N = 50
Peripheral Edema	2.5	1.4	13.9	19.5	36.0
Palpitation	0.8	1.4	0.0	2.4	12.0
Headache	12.4	11.3	11.1	18.7	28.0
Flushing	0.0	4.2	2.8	8.1	20.0

In addition, adverse experiences that occurred in 0.5 up to 1.5 percent of patients who received PLENDIL in all controlled clinical studies (listed in order of decreasing severity within each category) and serious adverse events that occurred at a lower rate or were found during marketing experience (those lower rate events are in italics) were: *Body as a Whole:* Facial edema, warm sensation; *Cardiovascular:* Tachycardia, *myocardial infarction, hypotension, syncope, angina pectoris,* arrhythmia; *Digestive:* Vomiting, dry mouth, flatulence; *Hematologic: Anemia; Musculoskeletal:* Arthralgia, arm pain, knee pain, leg pain, foot pain, hip pain, myalgia; *Nervous/Psychiatric:* Depression, anxiety disorders, insomnia, irritability, nervousness, somnolence; *Respiratory:* Bronchitis, influenza, sinusitis, dyspnea, epistaxis, respiratory infection, sneezing; *Skin:* Contusion, erythema, urticaria; *Urogenital:* Decreased libido, impotence, urinary frequency, urinary urgency, dysuria.

Felodipine, as an immediate release formulation, has also been studied as monotherapy in 680 patients with hypertension in U.S. and overseas controlled clinical studies. Other adverse experiences not listed above and with an incidence of 0.5 percent or greater include: *Body as a Whole:* Fatigue; *Digestive:* Gastrointestinal pain; *Musculoskeletal:* Arthritis, local weakness, neck pain, shoulder pain, ankle pain; *Nervous/Psychiatric:* Tremor; *Respiratory:* Rhinitis; *Skin:* Hyperhidrosis, pruritus; *Special Senses:* Blurred vision, tinnitus; *Urogenital:* Nocturia.

Gingival Hyperplasia: Gingival hyperplasia, usually mild, occurred in <0.5 percent of patients in controlled studies. This condition may be avoided or may regress with improved dental hygiene. (See PRECAUTIONS, *Information for Patients.*)

Clinical Laboratory Test Findings

Serum Electrolytes: No significant effects on serum electrolytes were observed during short- and long-term therapy (see CLINICAL PHARMACOLOGY, *Renal/Endocrine Effects*).

Serum Glucose: No significant effects on fasting serum glucose were observed in patients treated with PLENDIL in the U.S. controlled study.

Liver Enzymes: One of two episodes of elevated serum transaminases decreased once drug was discontinued in clinical studies; no follow-up was available for the other patient.

OVERDOSAGE

Oral doses of 240 mg/kg and 264 mg/kg in male and female mice, respectively and 2390 mg/kg and 2250 mg/kg in male and female rats, respectively, caused significant lethality.

In a suicide attempt, one patient took 150 mg felodipine together with 15 tablets each of atenolol and spironolactone and 20 tablets of nitrazepam. The patient's blood pressure and heart rate were normal on admission to hospital; he subsequently recovered without significant sequelae.

PLENDIL®
(Felodipine, MSD)
Extended-Release Tablets

Overdosage might be expected to cause excessive peripheral vasodilation with marked hypotension and possibly bradycardia.

If severe hypotension occurs, symptomatic treatment should be instituted. The patient should be placed supine with the legs elevated. The administration of intravenous fluids may be useful to treat hypotension due to overdosage with calcium antagonists. In case of accompanying bradycardia, atropine (0.5-1 mg) should be administered intravenously. Sympathomimetic drugs may also be given if the physician feels they are warranted.

It has not been established whether felodipine can be removed from the circulation by hemodialysis.

DOSAGE AND ADMINISTRATION

The recommended initial dose is 5 mg once a day. Therapy should be adjusted individually according to patient response, generally at intervals of not less than two weeks. The usual dosage range is 5-10 mg once daily. The maximum recommended daily dose is 20 mg once a day. That dose in clinical trials showed an increased blood pressure response but a large increase in the rate of peripheral edema and other vasodilatory adverse events (see ADVERSE REACTIONS). Modification of the recommended dosage is usually not required in patients with renal impairment.

PLENDIL should be swallowed whole and not crushed or chewed.

Use in the Elderly or Patients with Impaired Liver Function: Patients over 65 years of age or patients with impaired liver function, because they may develop higher plasma concentrations of felodipine, should have their blood pressure monitored closely during dosage adjustment (see PRECAUTIONS). In general, doses above 10 mg should not be considered in these patients.

HOW SUPPLIED

No. 3585 — Tablets PLENDIL, 5 mg, are light red-brown, round convex tablets, with code MSD 451 on one side and PLENDIL on the other. They are supplied as follows:

NDC 0006-0451-28 unit dose packages of 100
NDC 0006-0451-58 unit of use bottles of 100
NDC 0006-0451-31 unit of use bottles of 30.

No. 3586 — Tablets PLENDIL, 10 mg, are red-brown, round convex tablets, with code MSD 452 on one side and PLENDIL on the other. They are supplied as follows:

NDC 0006-0452-28 unit dose packages of 100
NDC 0006-0452-58 unit of use bottles of 100
NDC 0006-0452-31 unit of use bottles of 30.

Storage

Store below 30°C (86°F). Keep container tightly closed. Protect from light.

MERCK SHARP & DOHME, Division of Merck & Co., Inc.
West Point, Pa. 19486

A.H.F.S. Category: 24:04

Issued July 1991 DC7650202